DENTAL PHOTONICS

MJP PUBLISHERS

DENTAL PHOTONICS

S. MOHAN

Former Vice-Chancellor, PRIST University, Thanjavur

Former Senior Professor of Materials Science,
Asian Institute of Medicine, Science and Technology University,
Malaysia, Hawassa University, Ethiopia

Dean-Research, Vel Tech University, Chennai 600 062

MJP PUBLISHERS

Chennai New Delhi Tirunelveli

MJP PUBLISHERS

ISBN 978-81-8094-345-4

Printed and bound in India

MJP Publishers
No. 44, Nallathambi Street,
Triplicane,
Chennai- 600 005

MJP 259

Publisher : **C. Janarthanan**

Project Editor: **C. Ambica**

Preface

Lasers have been used in dentistry since 1963 for a variety of indications from tooth decay, gum disease, biopsy or lesion removal to teeth whitening. There is wide and continuous expansion of application of laser in dentistry. Laser can be a precise, effective and smarter way to perform many dental procedures. The lasers deliver energy in the form of light. Laser may act as a cutting tool when used in dental hard tissues. It can be used for "curing" a filling, which helps to strengthen the bond between the filling and the tooth. Laser acts as a heat source in bleaching and enhances the effect of Bleaching Agents. Further, Laser Facilitates the Wound Healing, help in the Diagnosis of Dental Caries, and it has other hard tissue applications including Endodontics. The Ability to Control Power output and the Duration of Exposure on the Tissue Improves the success of Dental Laser Applications. Modern Day Patients Expect A Comfortable Pain Free Treatment With High Safety. Lasers Have Added Benefits Of Sutureless Soft tissue treatment without anesthesia and infection with minimal bleeding and faster healing. Hence, it is essential for the dental practitioner and academicians to know the laser fundamentals with types, safety and applications of lasers. Keeping this in mind, the book has been written to cater to the needs of dental professionals. The leading scientists and dental academicians contributed for this volume. The book consists of 7 chapters. The first chapter deals with the basics of lasers. This chapter is written by Dr. S. Mohan which is the backbone for developing any laser. In the second chapter, Prof. S. Mohan describes various types of lasers with emphasis on dental lasers. The third chapter on laser light-tissue interaction is written elaborately by Dr. V. Arjunan and Dr. Sujin P. Jose, the knowledge of which is essential for applications of laser in dentistry. The chapter four on "Lasers in Dentistry" by Dr. Bikash Jyoti Borthakur and Dr. S. Mohan gives a bird's eye view on applications of lasers in dentistry in general. The next chapter on "Laser application in Conservative Dentistry and Endodontics" is written by senior dental academician

Dr. Bikash Jyoti Borthakur and it deals with conservative dentistry and endodontics. The chapter six on "Laser Applications in Prosthodontics" is written by expert dentists Dr. R. Shakila and Dr. L. Jeevanandham. The last chapter on laser safety is contributed by Dr. S. Mohan.

Dr.S.Mohan acknowledges his thanks to all the contributing co-authors for sharing their expertise in this volume. The author is also thankful to his beloved granddaughter P. Mithra who has shown a new life to him. Last but not the last, the author wishes to thank Mr. J.C. Pillai and Mr. C. Jana Pillai for their untiring effort, support and encouragement in bringing out this book involving two different areas of science.

PONDICHERRY, INDIA **S.MOHAN**

List of Contributors

Prof. Dr. S. Mohan, Ph.D, D.Sc,

Dean-Research, Vel Tech University,
Avadi, Chennai 600 062, India (smoh1947@rediffmail.com)

Dr. Bikash Jyoti Borthakur, M.D.S.,

Professor & Head, Dept. of Conservative Dentistry & Endodontics,
Mahatma Gandhi Postgraduate Institute of Dental Sciences,
Indira Nagar, Puducherry 605006 (Email:bicaus@rediffmail.com)

Dr. R. Shakila, M.D.S,

Associate Professor, Dept. of Prosthodontics,
Mahatma Gandhi Postgraduate Institute of Dental Sciences,
Indira Nagar, Puducherry-605006 (pranashakila@gmail.com)

Dr. L. Jeevanandam, M.D.S,

Associate Professor, Dept. of Prosthodontics,
Mahatma Gandhi Postgraduate Institute of Dental Sciences,
Indira Nagar, Puducherry-605006

Dr. V. Arjunan, Ph.D,

Associate Professor, Department of Chemistry,
Kanchi Mamunivar Centre for Post-Graduate Studies,
Puducherry 605 008, India (varjunftir@yahoo.com)

Dr. Sujin P.Jose, Ph.D,

Assistant Professor, School of Physics,
Madurai Kamaraj University,
Madurai 625 021, India (sujamku@gmail.com)

Contents

1

Basics of Lasers

Prof. Dr. S. Mohan

Vel Tech University, Chennai – 600 062

1.1 INTRODUCTION

what is light? light is a form of energy. light is a transverse electromagnetic energy. these are the spontaneous answers that one can expect. visible light which is a small part of the electromagnetic spectrum ranges between 400 and 700 nanometers. The optical portion of the spectrum consists of the infrared, the visible region and the ultraviolet. These are polychromatic and diverging radiations. The photonics technology is concerned with wavelength between 10 microns and 100 nanometers. photonics is nothing but the generation and harnessing of laser radiations.

λ 1m		10^{-3}m		10^{-6}m		10^{-9}m	10^{-12}m
	Radio	Microwave	Infrared	Visible light	Ultra violet	X-Ray	Gamma ray

Laser light is a manifestation of a particular interaction between charged particles and electromagnetic (EM) waves that requires understanding of quantization of energy of EM waves and energy of atoms. The important point in light, is brightness.

We mean that the bright source creates a greater intensity on the surface. The intensity on the surface depends on the intensity of the source and the spread of the light after it left the source. This spreading is known as divergence.

Laser is a device that generates a very intense beam of light. It usually converts one form of energy into optical energy. The word LASER is an acronym for Light Amplification by Stimulated Emission of Radiation. That is, laser is a light-emitting device with continuous feedback arrangement. It is a process of amplification and laser is a special form of light. It possesses several wavelengths ranging from ultraviolet to infrared. Hence, it is also called as UVLASER, IRLASER, free electron lasers, etc. Further it cannot be compared with the ionizing radiations such as X-rays and gamma rays. The different materials such as solids, liquids and gases produce characteristic wavelengths (colours) of light and hence we have different lasers with characteristic wavelengths. In addition to the intensity, several special features make lasers a unique source from the conventional light sources. As all the light rays in the beam are of the same colour, the light is very purely monochromatic. Perfectly monochromatic light cannot be produced even by a laser but laser light is many times more monochromatic than the light from any other source. They are extremely well-collimated. That is, it spreads out very little as it travels (high directionality). Laser has a high degree of coherence. That is, the waves in a laser beam are very nearly the same wavelength, the same direction and the same phase. These three properties make the light coherent. Coherence is the property of laser light that distinguishes it from all other types of light. Laser radiations are characterized by a high degree of ordering of the light (photons) than any other sources. The stimulated emission gives multiphoton of precisely the same wavelength whose wave patterns are perfectly in phase. This special kind of unique radiation is known as coherent radiation. Coherence is the most fundamental property of laser light and distinguishes it from other light sources. Thus, a laser may be defined as a source of coherent light. Laser exhibits spatial coherence as well as temporal coherence. Spatial coherence means that the light at the top of the beam is coherent with light at the bottom of the beam. On the other hand, temporal coherence means that the laser beam remains coherent for a long time as they move past at a given point. If a laser is more monochromatic, then it has greater temporal coherence.

1.2 LASER RADIATION

In general, laser is named after its active medium. To understand the laser emission, we should know something about energy levels. We know that most of the atoms (or molecules) are available in the ground state at room temperature. Yet, a very few atoms are also available in the higher energy state. The most important requirement for a laser action is that the medium should posses a large number of atoms in the higher energy state than in the ground state. This situation is known as population inversion.

Suppose if we supply energy to a medium, the atoms in the ground state absorb the energy and go to the higher energy state. This phenomenon is known as absorption. Ordinarily the atoms in the higher energy state spontaneously decay into ground state by emitting photons. These photons are out of phase with one another and this process is entirely random. Hence, the emitted light contains many different colours. That is, an incoherent light is emitted in this process. Examples of such light are the radiations received from the sun, light bulbs and the fire. On the other hand, if the electron in the higher energy state can be stimulated by another photon of precisely the same wavelength as the incident photon, we get a stimulated radiation. Here, the atom must be stimulated before it emits its stored energy (light). The induced and inducing photons have the same energy and they have identical direction of their momentum and identical polarization. That is, the secondary photon finds itself in the same state as the primary photon.

Prof. Albert Einstein conceived the idea of stimulated emission as early as 1900 during his research on photovoltaic mechanism and proposed the new radiation in 1918. Based on Einstein's theoretical prediction of stimulated emission in 1916, Schawlow and Townes proposed MASER (Microwave Amplification by Stimulated Emission of Radiation) emission around 1950. But it was Maiman who created the first solid-state laser (λ = 694.3 nm) in 1960 in a ruby rod. Hence, it is appropriate to recognize Dr. Albert Einstein as the father of laser (Figure 1.1).

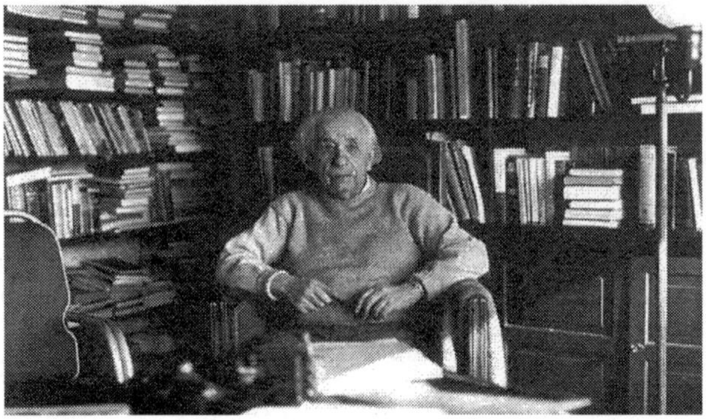

Figure 1.1 Albert Einstein (Courtesy: D. Samuel Gottesman Library)

Leon Goldman has done pioneering work in introducing laser technology in the field of medicine and he was responsible for promoting medical laser applications. Hence Leon Goldman is the father of lasers in medicine.

1.3 EINSTEIN COEFFICIENTS

According to Einstein, three optical properties occur in the formation of an atomic spectral line. The three optical processes are absorption, spontaneous emission and stimulated emission and they are associated with Einstein coefficients. These coefficients are the measure of the probability of the particular process.

Absorption is the process in which a photon is absorbed by electrons. This causes an electron to jump from a lower energy level to a higher energy level. The process is described by Einstein coefficient.

That is

$$B_{12}=B_{21} \tag{1.1}$$

$$A_{21} / B_{21} = (8\pi h\upsilon^3/C^3) \tag{1.2}$$

The above equation (1.1) shows that the spontaneous emission is predominant and laser is due to stimulated emission. Therefore, to achieve stimulated emission, population inversion is required. The laser action is possible only when $N_2 > N_1$. This non-equilibrium condition is known as population inversion. The equation (1.2) gives the relation between spontaneous and stimulated emission. This ratio is proportional to υ^3. The spontaneous emission increases with energy difference between two levels. The spontaneous and stimulated processes in a two level system is shown in Figure 1.2

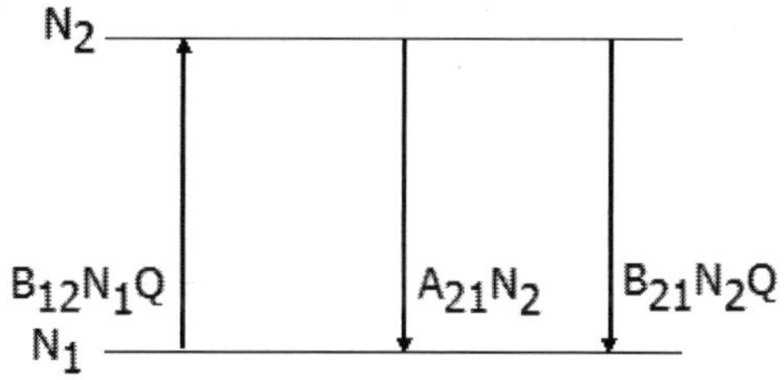

Figure 1.2 Spontaneous and stimulated processes in a two level system

Q is the radiation energy density and is equal to **N**hν, **N** being the number of photons of frequency ν per unit volume. For example, in an ordinary bulb having a filament temperature of about 5000 K and emitting radiation in the wavelength range of 0.6 micron corresponding to a frequency of 5×10^{14} Hz, the probability of stimulated emission is approximately one hundredth of that of the spontaneous emission. At lower temperatures, it can even be the orders less than this.

It is inferred that the ratio of the probability of spontaneous to stimulated light emission depends directly on the frequency of emission or inversely to the wavelength. Thus in the microwave region, stimulated emission is more probable than spontaneous and hence the early production of the maser. In the optical region, spontaneous emission is more likely than stimulated emission and this gets worse as we go into the UV and X-ray regions of the spectrum.

Before we discuss about the techniques of population inversion and laser action, let us remember the following salient points related to absorption, spontaneous emission and stimulated emission.

1.4 FEATURES OF ABSORPTION, SPONTANEOUS AND STIMULATED EMISSION

In case of *spontaneous emission* of a photon, the probability of its emission is inversely related to the average length of time an atom can reside in the upper level of the transition before it relaxes. This time is known as the *spontaneous lifetime* ($10^{-8} - 10^{-9}$ sec). The shorter the spontaneous lifetime, the greater is the probability that spontaneous emission will occur.

In certain materials, there are energy levels, which have the spontaneous lifetime of the order of microseconds to a few milliseconds. These levels are known as *metastable* levels. The probability of transitions involving metastable levels is relatively low.

When spontaneous emission decreases, the stimulated emission is increased. If an atom is excited into a metastable state it can stay there long enough for a photon of the correct frequency to arrive. Such a situation promotes stimulated emission at the expense of spontaneous emission.

In case of *stimulated emission*, atoms in an upper energy level can be triggered or stimulated in phase by an incoming photon of a specific energy. The incident photon must have an energy corresponding to the energy difference between the upper and lower states. The emitted photons have the same energy as incident photon. These photons are in phase with the triggering photon and also travel in its direction.

Stimulated processes like stimulated absorption or stimulated emission require incoming photons of the right frequency, whereas spontaneous emission can take place in the absence of incoming photon also.

Spontaneous emission is completely isotropic. On the other hand, stimulated processes have a built-in preference for emission in the direction of the incident flux of photons.

Whenever light is incident on the material, there is competition between absorption, spontaneous emission and stimulated emission processes. Under normal equilibrium conditions, the population of various levels is given by Boltzmann's relationship and thus N_2 will always be less than N_1. Further, stimulated photon emission is much less than the spontaneous photon emission and the absorption. For a system to work as a laser, the stimulated emission should exceed photon absorption. That is the two important conditions for laser mechanisms are:

(i) $N_2 > N_1$, i.e., Population Inversion.

(ii) It is clear that the value of Q (the radiation energy density which is equal to Nhν) should be as large as possible.

The first condition cannot be achieved under thermal equilibrium conditions. This implies that in order to create population inversion, one must look for non-thermal equilibrium system and thus the need for special laser materials.

1.5 LASER ACTIONS

The second condition that requires higher value of necessitates the use of an additional supply of large amount of energy of correct wavelength to excite the desired transition. The process is known as pumping. Various techniques include optical pumping, electrical pumping, chemical pumping and gas dynamic pumping, etc.

Although the population inversion is the primary condition, it is alone not sufficient for producing a laser. In addition to spontaneous emission, some losses arise for the emitted photons within the material. Hence, a geometry that can overcome these losses should be considered in such a way to achieve overall gain. This is possible with the help of optical cavity or resonator.

In laser, amplification arises as follows:

A large number of photons are produced in the excited state by pumping. If one of the atoms is emitted spontaneously, then the emitted photon would stimulate other atoms to emit. These emitted photons in turn stimulate other atoms for further emission which leads to amplification. Hence, the final photons emerge as an intense burst of coherent radiation.

The energy level diagram for three level laser and four level systems are shown in Figures 1.3 and 1.4, respectively.

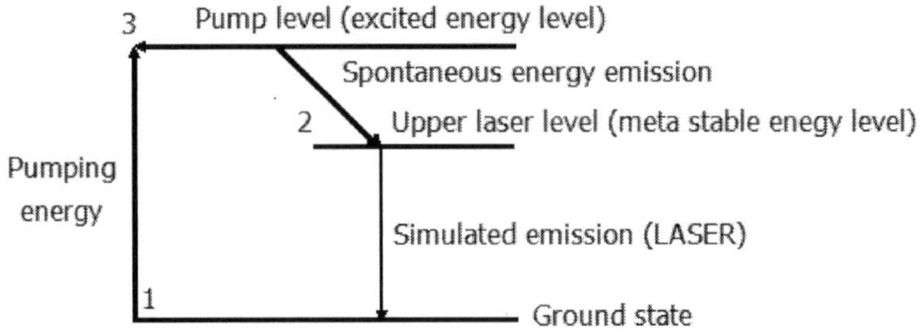

Figure 1.3 An energy level diagram for three level laser systems

In a three level laser system or a four level system, all the atoms are practically available in the ground state. The external energy excites them to a pump level and they spontaneously decay to upper laser level from there. In this process, the energy released is usually heat. The upper laser level has a long spontaneous life time and hence the atoms start accumulating at this level. This creates population inversion between this state and ground state. At lasing, the atoms at the upper level return to ground state by emitting photon which is nothing but a laser.

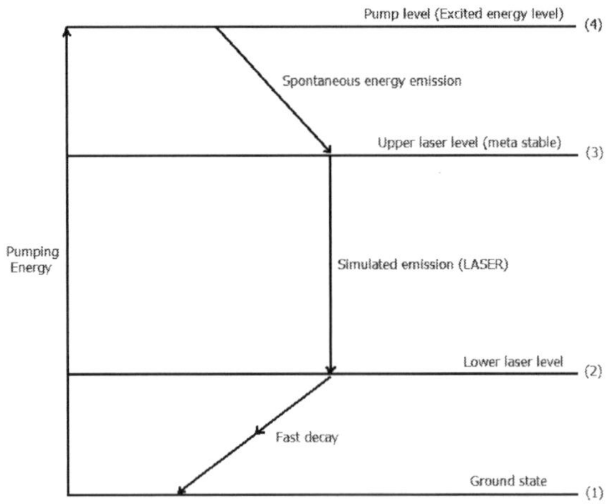

Figure 1.4 An energy level diagram for four level laser system

On the other hand in a four level laser, the material is pumped to level 4 which is a fast decaying level and the atoms decay rapidly to level 3, which is a metastable level. The stimulated emission takes place from level 3 to level 2 from where the atoms decay back to level 1. Four level lasers is an improvement on a system based on three level systems. In this case, the laser transition takes place between the third and second excited states. Since lower laser level 2 is a fast decaying level which ensures that it rapidly gets empty and as such always supports the population inversion condition. Energy appears as heat when the atoms decay from level 2 to level 1. Thereafter, the atoms decay and this energy appears as heat.

1.6 GAIN, SMALL SIGNAL GAIN AND SATURATION INTENSITY

For the development of lasers, one should understand, small signal gain, laser threshold, threshold pump power, saturation power and gain band width, etc.

1. *Small signal gain* of a laser medium is the optical gain obtained for a weak input signal which does not produce gain saturation.

2. The input power for the small signal gain is equal to the total cavity losses. This is defined as the *laser threshold* and the pump power for which the laser threshold is reached is called *threshold pump power*. One has to reach a compromise between high slope efficiency and low threshold power for optimization of the output.

3. Loop gain is defined as the total net gain that is obtained for a round trip transmission through the laser, after taking into account the losses.

4. The *saturation power* is defined as the power of that input signal which in the steady state produces a gain equal to one half of the value of its small signal gain.

5. *Gain bandwidth* is the finite range of frequencies in which gain is available.

1.7 IMPORTANCE OF SATURATION INTENSITY

The output of a laser depends on the energy stored in the laser material. The stored energy density (J/m^2) in a laser material is directly related to the pump energy and can also be modified by:

1. The overlap of the pump spectrum to the absorption spectrum of the material.
2. The intrinsic efficiency of the material.
3. Lifetime of upper excited energy laser level.
4. Saturation effects for very high pump energy densities.
5. The small signal gain g_o is directly proportional to population inversion, which in turn depends on the stored energy. Under small signal gain conditions, the maximum extractable energy is the product of stored energy E_{st} and area.
6. If E_{st} is far greater than the saturation energy, the degree of stimulated emission increases thereby reducing the population inversion and thus the reduction in output energy.
7. If E_{st} is less than the saturation energy, the degree of stimulated emission is less and thus the output energy is not optimum.
8. For efficient operation, lasers must operate with stored energy densities roughly comparable with their saturation energy density.

Saturation energy densities of common laser materials are as follows:

Nd:YAG:	0.7 J/cm2
Nd:Glass:	5 J/cm2
Ti:Sapphire:	0.9 J/cm2
Alexandrite:	30 J/cm2

Thus higher saturation energy density in Nd:Glass and Alexandrite suggest that higher output energies are possible in these materials.

1.8 THRESHOLD GAIN

Letter **'a'** in laser stands for amplification and obviously various aspects related to amplification is the key to laser generation. Amplification or optical gain in the laser medium is hindered by the cavity losses. The losses in the laser cavity prevent the available radiation to take part in the lasing process. The necessary condition for lasing is that the total gain in the system should be a little higher than all the losses. This input energy is referred to as laser threshold. Although lasing is supposed to start immediately (when the input energy reaches above laser threshold), useful, stable low noise performance and significant output can be obtained only much above laser threshold.

The cavity losses are due to:

1. Absorption and scattering losses in the gain medium, mirrors and other optical components.
2. Spontaneous emission losses.
3. Diffraction losses due to finite sizes of components.
4. Radiation losses through the output coupler, it being a partial reflector (unavoidable as partial reflectivity is essential for extracting the power from the laser).

In order to have a lower threshold and subsequent operation of an efficient laser system, one can employ high optical quality components with low absorption and scattering to reduce losses. Radiation losses through the output coupler can be minimized by optimizing its reflectivity. Thus one can achieve a low loss situation.

1.9 LASER COMPONENTS

The next question that comes to our mind is, how does a laser work? In general, all lasers consist of four components.

1. Active medium
2. Excitation mechanism
3. Feedback mechanism
4. Output coupler

1.9.1 Active Medium

The active medium is the main component of a laser. It may be a solid, liquid, gas or a semiconductor. Ruby, glass, alexandrite, neodymium:yttrium aluminium garnet (Nd: YAG) and holmium:yttrium aluminium garnet (Ho:YAG) are a few mediums for solid-state lasers. For electronic medium, semiconductors are used for producing diode lasers. For gas lasers, carbon dioxide, argon, krypton, helium–neon, helium–cadmium and rare earth halides (excited dimmers) are used as medium. Various kinds of dyes are used as medium for liquid lasers. Most lasers are based on 3 or 4 level energy systems, which depends on the lasing medium. These systems are shown in Figures 1.3 and 1.4.

1.9.2 Excitation Mechanisms

As a second step, we need energy source (power supply) to pump the active medium to achieve population inversion. Is it possible for the input energy to cause population inversion of atoms or molecules? We all know that the thermal energy can be used just to heat the atoms or molecules. Hence, it is not possible to achieve population inversion by this method.

Therefore one has to explore the other possibilities. One such possibility is just to remove some atoms out of the ground state energy level so that the ground state has less population than the higher energy level. Using this principle, the ***ammonia maser*** was built. Ammonia molecules were selectively filtered using electric field so that the remaining molecule exhibited population inversion. Unfortunately this method was not successful with optical masers (lasers).

The second possibility is ***electrical pumping***. This can be achieved by keeping the laser medium in the electron beam so that the electrons create a population inversion by transferring the energy to the atoms or molecules under collision. This technique is adopted in most of the high power gas lasers. The ***direct discharge*** is another technique of electrical pumping. As in the fluorescent lamp, electrical discharge can be affected in a tube containing the gaseous laser medium. A population inversion is created in the ions or atoms of the discharge when they absorb energy from the electrical current. The electrical discharge is used in common gas lasers such as carbon dioxide, argon, krypton, He–Ne and He–Cd lasers. This type of energizing the active medium is known as ***direct current method***.

One more method of creating population inversion is by using ***radio frequency energy***. The carbon dioxide lasers are partially energized by this technique. A sealed electrode tube of the gas is excited by an intense radio frequency field, creating a population inversion. These are known as ***sealed tube lasers***. They do not require external gas sources. It is self-contained within the laser resonator. Sometimes a small gas reservoir is also attached to the tube for laser's longer life. Ion lasers such as argon and krypton utilize an attached reservoir from which the tube must be periodically recharged manually. ***Carbon dioxide lasers*** are designed for flowing gas systems to several types of sealed systems.

Free space flowing gas systems are open glass tube with the mirrors at each end. When high voltage DC electricity is applied, it energizes the gas in the tube through the electrodes. After the emission of light radiation, the carbon dioxide molecule dissociates and contaminants are formed at the electrodes. Therefore, to sustain laser action, new gas must be continuously pumped which can be achieved by a vacuum system.

On the other hand, if we use a gas cylinder, it can last only for a few hours. Further, it is very expensive due to the escape of gas mixtures. When the gas is pumped through, the system is not a sealed tube. The scientific advancement has evolved microflow system which minimizes gas consumption. The main advantage in the ***gas ow system*** is that it operates indefinitely due to continuous fresh gas supply.

The most efficient carbon dioxide laser came into existence due to ***radio frequency waveguide*** lasers. These are sealed tube lasers which do not require costly gas tanks and are very quiet in operation. In these lasers, transverse radio frequency (high frequency electricity) signal across the tube is used to excite the gas instead of direct electrical excitation. One of the advantages of a high powered RF system is that high energy pulses may be developed in the super pulse mode on the laser which is very much greater than that attainable by direct electrical excitation. This produces higher average powers.

The next generation of carbon dioxide laser is ***free space sealed tube*** lasers. They have the main advantage of low operating costs due to the absence of external gas. These lasers use DC excitation just as the flowing systems. The difference is that they have a gas reservoir built right into the tube and use a special gas mixture. The large reservoir and catalysts reassociate the carbon dioxide molecules after it breaks apart so that it is continuously usable. These tubes will also have to be recharged after several thousand hours or three to five years or so.

Electrical pumping also creates a population inversion in semiconductor diode lasers—an important member in the laser family. When a current passes through the interface between *p*- and *n*-type semiconductors, it creates mobile charge carriers. If they are enough, it is possible to produce population inversion.

The third possibility is ***optical pumping***. In solid-state lasers like chromium-doped ruby and neodymium-doped YAG, the lasing atoms are embedded in a solid material. It is not possible to pump these lasers by an electrical current or an electron beam. Hence, they are optically pumped. The laser material is bombarded with photons whose energy corresponds to the energy difference between the ground level and the pump levels. The atoms in the ground state absorb energy from the pump photon and are excited to the pump bands.

The fourth possibility is the ***chemical energy*** to create a population inversion. Such lasers are known as chemical lasers in which two or more materials react, liberating energy and forming a new material. These new materials are treated with a built-in population inversion because many of its atoms or molecules have been excited by the chemical energy. Chemical lasers are capable of high powers but they are not very common. These lasers were developed by military for weapons in the past but today we have various types of lasers that are more appropriate for weapons.

For the sake of completeness, let us look into the fifth possibility of attaining population inversion. It is due to the ***nuclear particles***. Lasers have been pumped by nuclear particles, usually from nuclear bombs. The energy in the particles creates a population inversion in the laser medium and a pulse of laser output is obtained before the shock wave and other energy from the bombs destroys the laser. Such lasers may be useful to military applications alone.

Recently, we have a new family of lasers known as diode-pumped solid-state lasers which are commonly known as DPSSL. Here, semiconductor laser radiation is used as pump source for solid-state lasers. Combining non-linear crystals with this arrangement, it is possible to produce IR and deep UV lasers. It is also realized that this technology may very soon replace ion and gas lasers. Further, the cost of the lasers is very drastically reduced due to DPSSL.

Lastly, ***free electron lasers*** are pumped by high energy electrons. The output of a free electron laser is produced from electrons that are free. That is, the physics of a free electrons laser is much different from other lasers. There are no fixed energy levels for free electrons. Hence, laser wavelengths can be tuned. Although free electrons lasers are promising for future application, they are highly experimental and are in operation only in a few laboratories worldwide.

1.9.3 Feedback Mechanism

The next important aspect of lasers is the feedback mechanism (laser mirrors). The optical resonator is the device to amplify the light produced from stimulated emission. This device provides the necessary feedback for the laser to function. Optical resonator is nothing but a chamber or a laser tube (glass or quartz) that permits a series reflection of light waves back and forth at velocity of light between the two ends. Therefore the optical resonator essentially consists of a system of mirrors and the active medium. So, the photons are reflected back and forth for several times through the chamber stimulating more and more emission on each turn. Hence, the resonance builds in intensity and the light comes out through a partially transmissive mirror. The mirrors used at each end of the tube to form this resonator should be gently curved so that they tend to keep this light concentrated inside the resonator. One of the mirrors in the resonator is 100% reflective while the other mirror is partially reflective.

When photons bounce back and forth between the mirrors for a long period, the laser attains steady-state condition and a relatively constant power circulates between the mirrors. This circulating power is not absolutely constant. Interestingly, the power is lost when it hits the output mirror but the same is compensated while it is passing through gain medium. Mathematically, $P_{out} = \tau P_{cir}$ where τ is the transmission of the output mirror and P_{out} and P_{circ} are the output and circulating powers respectively.

By taking advantage of the partial reflective mirror, laser light emerges from the resonator. This is known as laser amplification which is used for optical gain. The process of stimulated emission starts amplification but the resonator plays an important role to increase the intensity to a high level. The emerging light from the partially coated mirror is the output beam from the laser. The partial reflective mirror varies from one type of laser to another but is usually somewhere between 1% and 50%.

Some lasers can produce easily 10 photons in a single pass and thus possesses enormous gain. These super radiant lasers do not need resonators. Nitrogen lasers sometimes operate in this way. Heavy metal vapour lasers such as copper and gold vapour also have such a high initial gain and hence they lase without mirrors. The mirror alignments which affect power output are much less critical in these type of systems. The actual gain in a laser resonator is in fact independent of the pump power. A few examples of optical resonators are:

1. A simple linear resonator,
2. A coupled linear resonator, and
3. A ring resonator.

Resonators used in lasers belong to the class of open resonators. They are considerably different from the cavity resonators used in the super high frequency (SHF) band. Fundamentally, an open resonator differs from a cavity resonator in two main aspects.

1. The conducting side walls are removed but the end face reflectors are retained. The end mirrors fix the resonator axis in space.
2. The dimensions of the resonator should be larger than the radiation wave length.

The quality factor Q of the resonator is defined as (assuming that only one mode exists) the ratio of energy stored in the cavity to the energy loss per radiation.

The smaller the losses in a resonator, the higher its Q. Further, the Q factor of a resonator is inversely proportional to the rate of decrease of field energy in the resonator.

Laser mirrors are coated with dielectric (cerium oxide) or metal layers. The manufacturing of laser mirrors are very complicated. The solid-state laser mirrors are formed on the specially prepared end faces of the active medium. In the case of gas lasers, resonator mirrors are usually mounted at both ends of the gas discharge tube with bellows.

Optical resonators give the direction for the emission of radiation. The process of stimulated emission just compensate for absorption only in this direction. That is, the resonator picks out a direction in space for which the losses are minimized and the condition for generation is satisfied.

It is also possible to add additional optical elements within the optical resonator to maintain selectively for photon states. A prism inside the resonator provides to select energy using the concept of dispersion of light.

The laser medium can be enclosed in a variety of resonator configurations.

1. Fabry–Perot configuration
2. Long radii mirror configuration
3. Concentric mirror configuration
4. Confocal configuration
5. Hemispherical configuration

The resonators, listed above are stable resonators wherein the beam is usually trapped inside and losses are only due to diffraction. That is, the light is concentrated near the axis of the resonator. If one traces the path of the ray of light between the mirrors of a stable resonator, the ray is eventually reflected back and forth towards the resonator axis by the mirrors. If at all the ray wants to escape, it has to pass through one of the mirrors. Hence, by saying "stable" we mean the trapping of rays between the mirrors. It is nothing to do with resonator's sensitivity to non-alignment.

On the other hand, in the unstable resonator, the light rays keep on moving away from the resonator axis until they miss the small convex mirror completely. The output beam from this resonator will have a doughnut-like shape with a hole in the middle caused by the shadow of the small mirror. It is also possible to construct unstable resonators without a hole in the central beam. The advantage of the unstable resonators is that they usually produce a large beam volume inside the gain medium so the beam can interact with more of the population inversion and thereby produce more output power. Unstable resonators sometimes produce more output than more conventional stable resonators. Unstable resonators are usually used only with high-power, pulsed gas and solid-state lasers. There are a number of important laser applications where the large diffraction losses in the unstable region are acceptable or even desirable.

A basic laser system can be depicted in Figure 1.5.

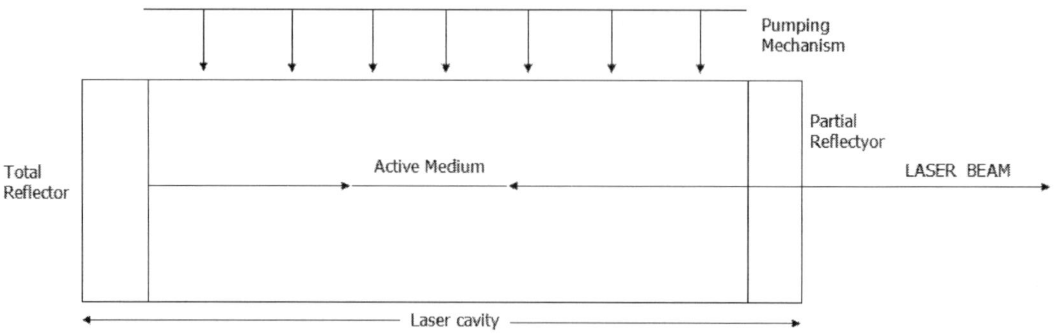

Figure 1.5 Basic laser systems

That is, for a laser production, the following features are essential.

(1) An active medium with a suitable set of energy levels to support laser action,

(2) A source of pumping energy in order to establish a population inversion and

(3) An optical cavity or resonator to introduce optical feedback and to maintain the gain of the system by overcoming all losses is essential.

1.9.4 Output Couplers

Output coupler is a partially reflecting dielectric mirror used in a laser cavity and they have reflectance in the range 40% to 70%. Laser Output Couplers are used as resonator mirrors for low, medium and high power lasers. The purpose of the output coupler is to divide an incident beam (monochromatic) into reflected and transmitted beams with the specified intensity ratio. They are coated with partial reflection coating (dielectric) on one side and anti-reflection coating on the other side. To optimize power and spatial profile of the laser beam, the output coupler and end mirror have optical surfaces with well-defined radii of curvature. Concave mirrors help to maintain TEM_{00} spatial mode within the resonator while wedged mirror deflect Fresnel reflection that could be amplified within resonator and form secondary (parasitic) pulse. The end mirror usually has reflectance of 99.5%. That is, the transmitted laser beam has low power.

1.10 RESONATOR MODES

The transverse and longitudinal are the two kinds of resonator modes. Resonator modes are the modes of an optical resonator (cavity). They are field distributions which reproduce themselves (apart from a possible loss of power) after one round trip. They can exist whether or not the resonator is geometrically stable but the mode properties of unstable resonators are fairly complicated.

The transverse spatial distribution of energy within the resonator leads to an understanding of how a laser beam propagates through space outside the resonator. Further, it will help to select the proper resonator mirrors to produce a laser beam of a given size and divergence.

Let us also see how the ***longitudinal*** spatial distribution of energy within a resonator affects the output beam from the laser.

Modes of laser resonators can differ significantly from those of an empty resonator because they are subject to transversely varying gain and loss. This gives rise to some deformation of the spatial shape and the modes are no longer mutually orthogonal. This leads to a set of adjoint modes, related to the actual resonator modes by some biorthogonality relations. This biorthogonal (non-normal) nature has a number of peculiar implications. For example, the total power circulating in the laser is no longer simply the sum of the powers propagating in the different modes. There are also effects on the laser noise.

Now, let us examine the shape of the ***transverse*** modes of a resonator.

The pattern inside the resonator moves out through the mirror and becomes the shape of the output beam. The beam can have number of profiles. The mode shapes can be created by forcing a resonator to oscillate in only one mode at a time. But the laser oscillating in many modes will not necessarily produce more power than one oscillating in a single mode because most of the available power must be divided among the oscillating modes. Each mode has a different designation. Incidentally, there is no strict code for deciding which subscript comes first. Writing either TEM_{61} or TEM_{16} are correct.

For many laser applications, it is important that the laser oscillate only in the TEM_{00} mode. The TEM_{00} mode is smaller in diameter than any other transverse mode.

Figure 1.6 The Shapes and intensity distributions of TEM_{00} laser mode (Courtesy:https://www.google.co.in/search?q=TEM00+-mode+figure&newwindow=1&tbm=isch&imgil=0hEUAukBjQ-6jHM%253A%253BDd86L95RD3bn1M%253Bhttp%25253A)

Higher order modes can be suppressed by placing an aperture inside the resonator. TEM_{11} mode occupies larger volume in the gain medium than TEM_{00} mode does. This mode interacts with more of the population inversion and extracts more power from the laser. For this reason, lasers oscillating in high order modes usually produce more power than similar lasers limited to TEM_{00} oscillation. Due to the importance of the TEM_{00} mode, it is also known as Gaussian mode, fundamental mode and diffraction limited mode.

1.11 LASER BANDWIDTH

In laser technology, laser bandwidth is also known as line width and spectral width. Physically it means the degree of monochromaticity of the laser output and bandwidth of a laser is an important parameter. If the temporal coherence of a laser is greater, then bandwidth is smaller. The optical Doppler effect, fuzzy energy levels, inhomogeneous broadening and homogeneous broadening are a few broadening mechanisms. Hence, laser bandwidth should be reduced. If the resonator provides wide-band feedback, then the bandwidth of the output will be as large as the bandwidth of the population inversion. But if the bandwidth of the feedback is reduced, the laser bandwidth is also reduced. In another technique, the intracavity prism reduces the bandwidth of resonator feedback and therefore the laser bandwidth. Instead of prism, an intracavity grating too does the same job. A birefringent filter is another device that reduces laser bandwidth by narrowing the bandwidth of the resonator's round-trip.

1.12 Q-SWITCHING AND GIANT PULSE

Q-switching is a novel and simple concept to generate giant laser pulse. Q-switching is another common term technically used to represent giant pulses. In Q-switching technique, the energy is stored in the population inversion until it attains a certain level. Subsequently, it is released very quickly as a giant pulse. In Q-switching lasers, all the energy comes out in a single giant pulse. This can be easily compared with storing water in a tank and then releasing the water suddenly. Is it possible to achieve this in laser?

In fact Q-switching is due to modulation of losses. This term describes the pulsing technique that produces peak powers of the order of 10 watts. These pulses have duration of only a few nanoseconds. Due to the short pulse width, the total energy of light emitted per pulse is very low—of the order of 3–10 millijoules.

1.13 WHY IT IS CALLED Q-SWITCHING OR Q-SPOILING?

The "Q" stands for the quality or quality factor of the resonator. Q-switching is also known as Q-spoiling or quality of the resonator. A high Q resonator possesses low loss. Basically, a resonator with a blocked mirror does not have very high Q. On the other hand, when the mirror is suddenly unblocked, the Q is switched from low to high. Hence, a Q-switched laser resonator can be switched from low quality to high quality and back. Q-switching is a technique whereby one controls the "Q" or feedback of the optical cavity. It generates short pulses of high peak power.

In Q-switching technique, stimulated emission plays an important role. That is, the Q-switch must switch the resonator from low Q to high Q to start the pulse but stimulated emission use up all the population inversion and terminate the pulse. In short, the laser lases until the population inversion is all gone but not until the Q-switch turns it off.

The duration of the pulse is not due to Q-switching but it depends mainly on how long the energy takes to get out the population inversion and out of the resonator itself. The pulse duration from Q-switched lasers range from nanosecond to femto (f) second. The pulse can be short as several nanoseconds from a high gain laser or several hundred nanoseconds from a low gain laser.

A high quality (high Q) resonator has low loss. Obviously, a resonator with an obstructed mirror is not a very high quality resonator. But, when the mirror is suddenly unblocked, the Q is switched from low to high. Thus a Q-switched laser is one whose resonator can be switched from low quality to high quality and back again. Therefore giant pulse lasers can be realised by controlling losses in the resonator. If these losses are sufficiently increased by some technique for a certain time, oscillation cannot develop. Consequently, the system of pumping builds a considerable overpopulation of the upper lasing level in active centers. If the losses are sharply brought down, the process of stimulated emission by the favoured photon states develops in a sudden manner and gives rise to a short light pulse with very high peak power.

All the lasers cannot be Q-switched. The life time of the upper laser level must be long enough so that energy does not leak out by spontaneous emission before the resonator Q is switched up, to stimulate a pulse. This is not the case for many types of lasers including ion lasers and dye lasers. The solid-state lasers such as YAG, glass or ruby can be made as Q-switched lasers.

In a typical continuous wave (CW) laser, one cannot operate with $\Delta N > (\Delta N)_{threshold}$. Therefore, the laser power will always be low. But, in a Q-switch laser, one prevents laser oscillation, thereby allowing ΔN to grow larger than $(\Delta N)_{threshold}$. The laser is then "turned on" and power is rapidly extracted. A typical arrangement to generate giant pulse is shown in Figure 1.7.

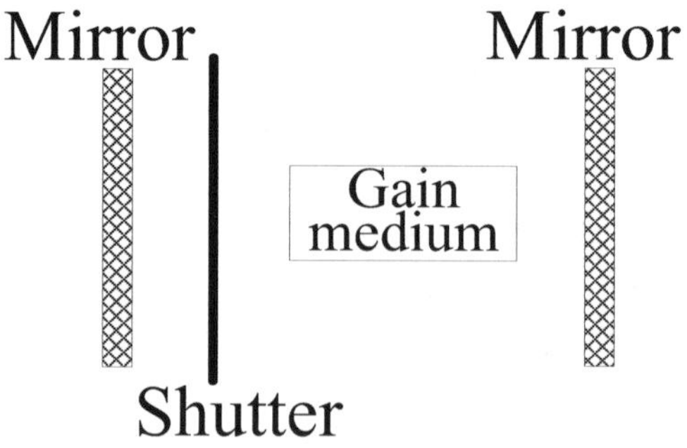

Figure 1.7 A typical arrangement to produce giant pulse

Although Q-switching does not produce the shortest pulses available (mode-locking does that), it has several advantages.

1. It is inexpensive.
2. It is easy to implement.
3. It is efficient in extracting energy stored in upper laser level.

In order to control the losses in a resonator, four types of Q-switching are used in lasers.

Table 1.1 Types of Q-switching used in lasers

Sl.No	Mechanism	Process
1	Mechanical Q-switches	Active Q-switch—move a mirror to switch the resonator Q
2	Acousto-optic Q-switches	Active Q-switch—diffraction reduces feedback from a resonator mirror
3	Electro-optic Q-switches	Active Q-switch—polarization prevents light from returning from a mirror
4	Dye (chemical) Q-switches	Passive Q-switch—absorbs the light and bleaches the dye

The advantages and disadvantages of electro-optic switches are as follows:

Advantages

1. They are faster than mechanical switches.
2. They are not noisy.
3. They do not produce any vibrations.
4. They are not very costly.

Disadvantages

1. Their construction as well as explanation is slightly difficult.

2. Although they are faster than mechanical switches, they are slower than acousto-optic switches.

3. Voltage need for electro-optic crystal can be considered its disadvantage.

The advantages and disadvantages of acousto-optic switches are as follows:

Advantages

1. Q-switch is very fast with acousto-optic system. It is possible to produce laser pulses at the rate of 25000 pulses per second when an acousto-optic Q-switch is used in conjunction with continuous laser pumping system.

2. These switches do not produce noise during their operation.

3. Use of crystal is advantageous.

4. Acousto-optic devices have proved to be the most useful type for Nd:YAG lasers. The voltage required for operation of an electro-optic device increases with wavelength (a disadvantage for infrared applications). Bleachable dyes for Q-switching in the infrared are less developed than those for use in the visible. Thus acousto-optic devices are most useful for Nd:YAG Q-switching.

Disadvantages

1. Radio frequency (RF) generator is required to produce ultrasonic waves.

2. The cost of acousto-optic switches are more than mechanical switches.

The advantages of chemical Q-switches are:

In chemical Q-switches, organic dye goes through its bleaching cycle vary rapidly. That is why these can also be used to mode-lock a laser.

1. The chemical Q-switches are not noisy.

2. These types of switches do not produce any vibrations.

If the Q-switching occurs rapidly for emission of multiple pulses, the peak power of each pulse is less than that of single pulses of lower frequencies but is still much higher than a gated pulse. The potassium titanyl phosphate crystal for instance will Q-switch the laser beam at over 25,000 times per second.

1.14 SUPERPULSE

Superpulse is found on many carbon dioxide lasers and they are usually called as superpulse, varipulse or megapulse. This pulse on CO_2 lasers usually produces a train of pulses from 250 to 500 watts with a maximum peak power per pulse at a rate of 300–1000 times per second. This rate is so fast that it appears to be continuous but the pulse can be picked up as an audible sound as and when the focused beam hits the target. Further, the total delivered energy is not as high as the 500 watt pulse but it comes to only 75 millijoules per pulse. This is the average power of the CO_2 lasers. The maximum average power in a superpulse will always be substantially lower than the maximum power available in continuous mode. Most lasers produce approximately one-third of the high power in super pulse in comparison with a continuous wave mode. High power lasers, such as 80–100 watts allow for superpulsing approximately 25–35 watts average power. Lower power lasers often produce maximum superpulsing of only 10–20 watts average power. These lower energies per pulse and average powers are useful for cutting but they are insufficient for vaporizing large areas. Hence, the higher powers of a continuous wave mode are useful for vaporization.

An exception is the superpulse mode on some RF-excited CO_2 lasers which are known as ultrapulse. These lasers produce such high energies per pulse so that the average power is not sacrificed. In fact, it can produce average ultrapulse powers as high as the maximum CW power on the laser.

1.15 MODE-LOCKING

Mode-locking is a technique to produce ultrashort pulses from lasers and such lasers are known as *mode-locked lasers*. Mode-locking is all about gain or loss. The highest pulse frequency and the shortest pulse are obtained by mode-locking a laser. The shortest pulse of light that have ever been generated come from mode-locked lasers.

The technique of mode-locking is based on an active modulation of the intra-cavity losses or the round-trip phase change. In mode-locked lasers, the laser resonator contains either an active element such as an optical modulator or a nonlinear passive element namely a saturable absorber which causes the formation of an ultrashort pulse circulating in the laser resonator.

The duration of a Q-switched laser pulse varies from several hundred nanoseconds to several nanoseconds depending on the laser parameters. The cavity dumped laser pulse is shorter than nanoseconds. But a mode-locked pulse from a dye laser can be shorter than a picosecond. Mode-locked lasers can be operated either with a pulsed or CW pump.

Any type of laser can be mode-locked, even a one that is already been Q-switched or cavity dumped. In fact, some lasers are simultaneously Q-switched, cavity damped and mode-locked. A mode-locked pulse from a dye laser can be shorter than a picosecond. The working of a mode-locked laser can be understood either by time domain or by frequency domain.

The duration of the mode-locked pulses depends on laser's gain bandwidth and effectiveness of the mode-locking modulator (its modulation depth). The greater the laser's bandwidth, the shorter the mode-locked pulses. (Nd:YAG lasers possess relatively narrow bandwidths and hence produce *mode-locked* pulses of 30–60 ps in duration). Electro-optic modulators, acousto-optic modulators and dye cells are used to mode-lock lasers. The longitudinal modes of the resonator are locked together in phase when we mode-lock a laser. This is also referred to as phase locking.

Mode-locked lasers do not usually have very high peak power. However, they are used to get very short pulses. Although mode-locked lasers are usually not used in the fiber optic, terrestrial communication links are now being integrated into many telephone systems. They are used by the military for communication among space craft and with submarines. The mode-locked lasers are also used in ranging and in spectroscopic tools to investigate very fast phenomena. Mode-locking can be combined with any other techniques to produce lasers or it can be used by itself to produce an unending train of mode-locked pulses.

1.15.1 Difference Between Mode-Locking and Q-Switching

Mode-locking is a technique for producing periodic, high power, short duration laser pulses. Depending on the properties of the laser, these pulses may be of extremely brief duration, as short as a few femto seconds.

Major difference between Q-switching and mode-locking is as follows. Before generation of the output pulse the energy is stored in the intra-cavity light field in mode-locking whereas in case of Q-switching it is stored in the gain medium. The most important advantage of mode-locking is that this energy can be extracted within just one round-trip time and is independent of the time required for building up the intra-cavity power. Therefore, the pulse duration achievable is more or less determined by the resonator length (provided that the switching time of the modulator is not longer than the resonator round-trip time) and is decoupled from the laser gain. This means that even for very high pulse repetition rates, e.g., several megahertz, pulse durations of a few nanoseconds are still achievable. In case of mode-locking, pulsed laser action is attained by coupling together the modes of lasers and locking their phases to each other.

In case of Q-switching, the number of radiation transits through the switch whether active or passive, are usually few. But in case of mode-locking the radiation transits large number of times through the switch. In case of Q-switching, the laser output is turned off by increasing the resonator loss, i.e., by spoiling the resonator quality factor Q periodically with the help of a modulated absorber inside the resonator. Thus Q-switching is loss switching. When the losses are reduced during the "on" times, the large accumulated population difference is released and hence generates short intense pulses of light. The most commonly used mode-locked lasers are given in Table 1.2.

Table 1.2 Commonly used mode-locked lasers

Active medium	Modulator	Mode-locking operation	Pulse width
Gas Lasers			
He–Ne	Quartz–AM	CW	1 ns

He–Ne	Neon cell–SA	CW	350 ps
Ar	Quartz–AM	CW	150 ps
CO_2 (low pressure)	SF–SA	CW	10–20 ns
CO_2	Ge–AM	CW	10–20 ns
CO_2 (TEA)	Ge–AM	Pulsed	1ns
CO_2 (TEA)	SF –SA	Pulsed	1 ns
Solid-state lasers			
Nd:YAG	Quartz–AM	CW	100 ps
Nd:YAG	LinBO–EOM	Pulsed	40 ps
Nd:glass	Kodak–9860 SA	Pulsed	5 ps
GaAs	SA	CW	5 ps
Liquid (Dye lasers)			
Rhodamine 6G	DODCI–SA	Flash-pumped	1 ps
Rhodamine 6G	Sync. pump	CW, Ar-pumped	0.5 ps

AM–Acousto-optic modulator, SA–Saturable absorber
EOM–Electro-optic modulator, DODCI–3, 3-Diethyloxydicarbo cyanine iodide

1.16 BASIC MODES OF LASER OPERATION

Laser oscillation can be broadly classified under three categories.

1. Continuous oscillation,
2. Pulsed oscillation, and
3. Pulsed mode with controlled losses (Q-switching lasers).

The gas lasers give a continuous mode while pulsed modes are mostly seen in solid lasers. In continuous wave lasers, the light beam is emitted with constant power.

That means, this mode requires a continuous steady-state pumping of the active medium. This can be achieved by continuously operating optical pumping or by a steady-state discharge in a gas. The cross section of the laser beam in these lasers is always lesser than the cross section of the resonator.

In pulsed free oscillation, the radiation comes out in the form of periodic light pulses from 1 to 10 seconds long at a frequency of 10 Hz to 10 kHz. The pulsed laser is due to the pulsed operation of the pumping system, viz., a flash lamp. In solid-state lasers, the laser beam cross section is equal to the cross section of the active medium. In pulsed mode oscillation, we achieve a considerable concentration of light energy. In these lasers we get a substantial power output within short time intervals. The concentration of light energy reaches a maximum in the giant pulse mode of oscillation.

Continuous wave (CW) generally refers to a steady-state power output from the laser. Although medical lasers offer a choice of operating modes to include continuous and pulsed mode, most medical lasers work in the CW mode.

In a pulsed laser, a true laser pulse can compress the power output of the laser tube and deliver a very high peak power of energy during the pulse but cannot maintain these high powers in a steady state. It delivers peak powers which are generally not attainable when operating with a CW beam. Pulsing includes Q-switching, mode-locking, superpulsing and flash lamp pulsing techniques. With the exception of superpulse, most pulsing is designed into the laser.

Some lasers deliver their energy solely as pulsed energy and many CO_2 lasers additionally offer a superpulse mode. Timer on the CW beam is most commonly referred to as gated pulse and it is common on CO_2 lasers.

True laser pulses, which are different, may also be emitted in this timed fashion. Most of the CO_2 lasers offer an option for a repeat pulse which is a very useful feature on CO_2 lasers.

1.17 ULTRASHORT PULSES

When the lamp flashes, the electro-optic Q-switch is in its transmission mode. Therefore, light passes through Pockels cell without any polarization rotation. When the round-trip gain becomes equal to the round-trip loss, the laser begins lasing. The photons start bouncing back and forth between the mirrors. Due to 100% reflectance mirror, the circulating power increases to a very high level. When the maximum intracavity circulating power has been obtained, a voltage is applied to the Pockels cell. The cell rotates the polarization of light passing through it and the polarizer ejects all the light in a cavity-dumped pulse. Cavity dumping is a general technique that can be used with advantage whether the laser be mode-locked or CW or Q-switched. For pulsed, mode-locked lasers, cavity dumping is usually carried out at the time when the intracavity mode-locked pulse reaches its maximum value. In this way, a single ultrashort pulse of high intensity comes out of the laser cavity.

For generating ultrashort pulses, one needs 1) laser medium with broad spectrum, 2) fast saturable absorber, and 3) proper dispersion compensation.

Ultrashort pulses, tunable from the visible to mid-infrared are useful for many applications such as pulse propagation in optical fibers, carrier dynamic studies in semiconductors, in time-resolved relaxation dynamics and the observation of transient chemical species. This is achieved due to the concept of mode locking in the last four decades. A widely tunable ultrashort pulse laser sources are also available for the investigation of optical properties (including second and third order non-linear properties) of both organic and inorganic materials. Several techniques exist to generate tunable picosecond pulses. Synchronously mode-locked continuous-wave colour center lasers directly generate picosecond pulses in the infrared but their tunability (for a given center type and host material) is limited and these systems generally suffer from a photo bleaching effect which results in fading and poor reliability. On the other hand, synchronously mode-locked dye lasers are reliable and tunable sources. The recent progress in the development of efficient infrared dyes has extended the laser wavelengths coverage to about 1.3 fm.

In recent years, enormous advances have been made in the generation of ultrashort pulses. It is possible to carry out a wide range of measurements within the time scale of 10^{-10} s (pico second) and 10^{-15} s (femto second). In order to derive the ultrashort pulse from a laser, the fluorescence or gain bandwidth of the amplifier must be sufficiently broad to support the pulse. Mode-locking techniques have been used in the last two decades to generate ultrashort pulses. During that time, various refinements to the technique have led to the development of laser systems capable of operating in the femto second range.

1.18 ENERGY CONCEPTS

Laser power is expressed in milliwatts (mW) to megawatts (MW) to gigawatts (GW). There is a considerable difference between small m and capital M. This indicates whether the laser is a low power laser or a high power laser. Power in watts is a measure of the rate of energy delivery in joules/second. To determine peak power of a laser pulse, energy delivered is divided by the required time. For example, if 200 millijoules is delivered in 200 microseconds, the peak power is 1000 watts.

Power density is the important factor in the effective operation of any laser. It is synonymous with irradiance. It determines the laser's ability to vaporize, excise and coagulate various tissues of the body. It describes the intensity of light in terms of power per unit area. Power density is expressed in watts/cm. The surface area of the spot (spot size controlled by the surgeon) and the total power of the laser in watts determine the power density. If the spot radius is in millimeters, then power density helps in determining the rate of tissue removal and creates the perception of eye-hand coordination of the physician. A common misconception is that power alone determines the coordination required to avoid perforations or shredding of tissue with the laser. Power density over a spot determines the rate of tissue removal within that spot. One can effectively change the size of the spot with which one is working, without changing the overall rate of tissue removal (power density) within the spot by varying spot size and power. The larger the spot, the greater is the power required to maintain the same power density. At extremes, a very low power density is very easy to control by the surgeon but it burns tissue excessively. On the contrary, a very high power density produces a very clean tissue effect but it is very hard to control by the surgeon. When vaporizing or debulking tissue, spot sizes are made easier so that the total time required to burn the tissue can be considerably reduced.

The total light energy is described by the unit Joule. Laser pulses are measured in joules (1 Joule = 1 watt second). Therefore the total energy delivered depends upon the power and the duration of the laser source. That is, longer the light is delivered or higher the power, the total energy delivered is more. Joules describes the total energy delivered but does not indicate how concentrated is this light dose. For example, surgical Nd:YAG and ophthalmic lasers have joules read out while carbon dioxide lasers do not have joules read out. The rate of energy delivery is described by flux. For example, 100 joules can be delivered in 1 second by 100 watts or in 100 seconds by one watt. 100 watts per second is a higher flux.

Combining the concept of rate of delivery with that of power density leads to the concept of 'fluence'. The unit of fluence is joules/cm. Fluence is also known as radiant exposure. Fluence is an energy concept which considers both radiant pressure and power density from the surface and exposure from all other directions. In short, high energy delivery in quicker phase is represented by fluence. When the fluence is very high, it has very precise thermal effect on tissues. Due to very high peak power, laser pulse with short period of exposure, minimizes or eliminates any unwanted heat conduction to adjacent tissues. Due to this, superpulsing CO_2 laser gives a clear cutting effect. The pulsed laser of this type is also used to make birth marks and similar lesions which minimize any unwanted burning effects of the laser. The high fluence pulsed laser energy creates non-linear effects. These are generally acoustical shock waves not associated with direct tissue heating. A Nd:YAG pulsed laser of tens of millions of watts within a few nanoseconds can create the cold cutting sparks used inside the eye to cut membranes. A little lesser power than the above laser is a pulsed dye laser which has high fluence can create shock waves. In combination with fiber, the shock waves can destroy the kidney stones also.

Even when a low power laser is left in a place for a considerable time, the thermal conduction of adjacent tissues is very extensive. It is very important to visualize this spread of heat during any laser procedure. The excess tissue damage is proportional to the time the beam is applied. It does not depend on the total power. That is why surgeons should choose the high power density laser. Further he/she can control the time of exposure to perform the jobs quietly and restrict the spread of damage.

This principle applies only where power density is greater than 1000 watts/cm at the tissue. Let us not be under the impression that significantly high power densities, achieved by using very small spots with low power lasers will achieve satisfactory surgical results for vaporization. In order to debulk or vaporize large volume of tissues, the spot must be broadening, approximately to the size of a pencil eraser. This allows for more uniform, smooth vaporization of tissues but requires higher total power to compensate for the dilution of power density. If one tries to debulk a mass with a pinpoint spot size and high power densities, it will create uneven ridges, furrows, bleeding and is generally unsatisfactory. An elegant technical solution to the problems is to use a random electronic scanner with these focused beams. The speed of the scan eliminates the problems of high power density spots while retaining the clean tissue effects. This is one way of achieving high fluence with a CW beam. This gives a char-free clean tissue vaporization. While selecting a laser apparatus, one has to pay attention towards the power density which is an important parameter. Hence, the higher the power capabilities of the laser, the greater are its applications and future flexibility.

For example, CO_2 laser with power range of 50–60 watts is more versatile for all specialists. Although the higher powers of CO_2 lasers are available, they are very costly and may not find many applications. One aspect of 50–60 watts CO_2 laser is its potential limitations which may pose on pulsed average power such as superpulse. The other advantage of high power CO_2 lasers ranging from 60 watts to 100 watts is that the average power of the superpulse is also in the useful range. In the recent years, CO_2 lasers have become out-dated and in its place DPSSL (Nd:YAG, KTP lasers) play an important role in the surgeon's hands.

1.19 IMPACT SIZE AND SPOT SIZE

The actual size of the incision width made by the laser on the object is known as impact size. When the laser beam is focused with the help of a lens, it is known as spot size. Spot size of the laser is an important factor which controls the power density.

The spot size depends on:

1. *Focal length of the lens* Short focal length of the lens produces smaller spots.
2. *Diameter of the incident beam into the lens* When the beam is larger, the spot size is smaller. This is inherent in the laser design.
3. *Wavelength of the light* When wavelengths of the laser beam are shorter, the spot sizes are smaller.
4. *TEM of the beam* Transverse electromagnetic mode, i.e., the TEM_{00} mode, produces the smallest spots.
5. *Delivery system* Fibers control spot size in a manner different from the focused beams. Spot diverges continuously from the fiber.

Lenses are interchangeable and therefore spot size can be controlled. The smaller the focal length of the laser lens, the smaller will be the spot and hence higher power density. For example, in a CO_2 laser unit, 400 mm lens gives 0.8 mm spot size; 300 mm lens gives 0.6 mm spot size; 200 mm lens gives 0.4 mm spot size and 125 mm lens gives 0.2 mm spot size.

The spot size of the focused beam is determined by the size, shape and colour of the beam as it enters a lens. The spot size of a laser is an entirely different thing from the impact size.

The spot size is a mathematical measurement whereas the impact size relates the active size of the crater (or incision width) left by the laser. Keeping spot size the same, the impact size will increase when the beam is applied longer to the site. The edges of the beam are longer to create an effect which increases its width.

The wavelength of the light also determines how small the spot may be focused. That is, when the wavelength is smaller, the spot size is smaller keeping all things equal. For example, an argon ion laser produces a much smaller spot than a carbon dioxide laser. However, the laser is chosen for its specific effects on tissues and delivery mechanism rather than for its spot size abilities. The mode refers to the distortion of power over the spot size area and determines the precision of the operative spot. The term used to describe this is transverse electromagnetic mode (TEM). The fundamental mode TEM shows an even power distribution over the spot so that most of the power is at the center and there are no hot or cold spots. A look at the power distribution reveals a cone-shaped pattern. The spot is brightest in the center and faded towards the edges. This mode can produce very fine spots.

Because the impact size of the beam on the tissue is a function of tissue heating, time is very important as spot size determines the actual impact size. The longer the beam is on, the more the heat builds up around the blurred fizzy edges of the spot and wider the impact. When the light is not distributed in this fundamental manner, it is said to be in multimode distribution. This can occur in many different patterns. But common mode in some older surgical lasers is the TEM_{01} mode. It has a cold spot in the center and it is also known as doughnut mode. It is not possible to focus this mode to a fine spot as TEM_{00} mode.

For example, a 400 mm lens and TEM_{00} beam would focus to 0.8 mm spot while the same lens with TEM_{01} would focus to 2.00 mm spot. High-power output of carbon dioxide laser changes the mode structure at the beginning of lasing. A high-power setting, viz., 80–100 watts used in timed pulses of around 0.1 seconds tends to create multimode beams and one sees the resulting beam in doughnut shape.

References

1. Jeff Hecht. *The laser guidebook*. McGraw-Hill, New York, 1986.

2. Orazio Svelto. 1989. *Principles of lasers*. Ed by David C. Hanna, Plenum New York.

3. *Laser handbook*. 1972. Ed. by F.T. Arecchi and E.O. Schulz-Dubois. North-Holland Pub. Co, Amsterdam and American Elsevier Pub. Co., New York.

4. Karl F. Renk. 2012. *Basics of Laser Physics*. Ringer Science & Business Media.

5. William T. Silfvast. 2004. *Laser Fundamentals*. Cambridge University Press.

6. K. Thyagarajan and Ajoy Ghatak. 2010. *Lasers: Fundamentals and Applications*. Springer Science & .Business Media.

2

Dental Lasers

Prof. Dr. S. Mohan

Vel Tech University, Chennai-600 062.

2.1 INTRODUCTION

So far we have seen the various principles employed in lasers. But we have not mentioned the laser types used in dentistry. Today, we are familiar with lasers such as helium-neon and diode lasers as bar code reader in shops, supermarkets, at home CD players, laser printers and in alignment activities. The number of laser systems in use today differ in active medium and in pumping methods. The following is a brief list of lasers used in dental applications. Lasers are an alternative to conventional surgery. They are also known as optical scalpel or light scalpel. The main advantage in usage of lasers is due to its comfort, cool, no fear, no cut and no sew. The common dental lasers on the electromagnetic spectrum are frequency doubled alexandrite, argon, He-Ne, Nd:YAG, Ho:YAG, Er:YAG, Er,Cr:YSGG, Nd:YAG, diode (InGaAs and AlGaAs) and CO_2. Each type of laser has specific biological effects and procedures associated with them. A thorough understanding of each of these lasers is necessary for clinicians using lasers in their practice. The properties of dental lasers are listed in Table 2.1.

Table 2.1 Dental Lasers

Lasers	**Wavelength in nm**	**Applications**
Frequency doubled alexandrite	377 nm	Periodontal treatment
Neodymium:YAG Nd:YAG	1318 (mid-IR)	Tissue welding (fusion), soft tissue desensitization, analgesia, endodontics, tissue cutting, intraoral soft tissue procedures, used for adjunctive periodontal procedures, tooth whitening, photo bio-modulation, soft tissue
Ho:YAG	2100	Vaporize, ablate and coagulate soft tissues and extremely hard materials
Er,Cr:YSGG	2780	Deep thermal penetration in tooth structure; Periodontal treatment
Diode lasers InGaAs AlGaAs	910-980 nm 750-880	Tissue cutting, intraoral soft tissue procedures, used for adjunctive periodontal procedures, tooth whitening, photo bio-modulation, soft tissue, periodontics
Erbium YAG Er:YAG	2940 (mid-IR)	Bone cutting and drilling; several dental procedures, hard tissue
Carbon-di-oxide	10600 (far-IR)	Incisional and excisional biopsies, frenectomy, gingivectomy, pre-prosthetic procedures, soft tissues, dentin desensitization.
Argon laser	488, 514.5	Curing, soft tissue, desensitization.

We will examine the above types of lasers in the following sections.

2.2 SOLID-STATE LASERS

Solid-state lasers are made by a crystal or a glass with small amount of doping such that the upper laser level is optically pumped by a suitable light source. There is another class of laser using a solid as active medium which are becoming more and more important. It is a semiconductor crystal, usually with one or more junctions and pumping is achieved by injecting a current in the crystal. Today SSLs are still one of the most important classes of lasers, both in industrial and medical applications. The only competitor in average power is the CO_2 laser. In medical applications, the possibility of transporting the laser beam by a thin optical fibre paves the way for easy surgery. In recent years the pumping mechanism is done not by flash lamps but by semiconductor lasers. Hence, we have a new class of lasers pumped by diodes. They are known as *diode-pumped solid-state lasers.*

2.2.1 561 nm DPSS LASER

The recent DPSS laser with yellow output at 561 nm (10 mW) from Melles Griot is an ideal excitation wavelength for biomedical fluorescence. The laser is pumped by a 1-W single stripe diode laser. It is expected to serve for 20,000 hours of operation.

2.2.2 DEVELOPMENTS IN DIODE-PUMPED SOLID-STATE LASERS

The recent advances in diode-pumped solid-state lasers (DPSSL) made a revolution in laser physics. DPSS lasers in many ways approach the ideal output power, beam quality and repeatability to those of gas lasers but their efficiency and size are more like those of semiconductor diode lasers. Although the initial cost of a DPSSL and an ion laser are comparable, annual operating cost of the DPSS system is significantly less because of its operating lifetime of nearly 10,000 hours. With modern InGaAs diode pumps, Yb:YAG lasers have been intensively developed and today we have successful Yb:DPSSLs. Yb-based lasers are said to operate in a "quasi three level" laser scheme. Beyond Yb:YAG, attempt has been made to achieve Yb-doped crystals with highly favourable spectroscopic properties. The nomenclature for new Yb-doped laser materials are given in Table 2.2.

Table 2.2 Nomenclature for new Yb-doped laser materials

DPSSL	Diode-pumped solid-state laser
YAG	$Y_3Al_3O_{12}$
FAP	$Ca_5(PO_4)_3F$
S-FAP	$Sr_5(PO_4)_3F$
KGW	$KGd(WO_4)_2$
KYW	$KY(WO_4)_2$
BCBF	$BaCaBO_3F$
CAS	$Ca_2Al_2SiO_7$
LNB	$LiNbO_3$
LTA	$LiTaO_3$
YCOB	$YCa_4O(BO_3)_3$

Subsequently materials science research yielded several Yb-doped crystals including hosts, which are as follows:

LiNbO-(LNB)
$Ca_2Al_2SiO_7$-(CAS)
$BaCaBO_3F$-(BCBF)
$SrLaGaO_4$
$SrLaGa_3O_7$
$KY(WO_4)$-(KYW)
$KGa(WO_4)_2$- (KGW)
$CuGaS_2$
$AgGaSe_2$
$AgGaS_2$
LiTaO-(LTA)
$YCa_4O(BO_3)_3$-(YCOB)

Yb-doped crystal DPSSLs continue to advance in performance using well-developed Yb:YAG crystal and developing Yb-doped fluoroapatite crystals. Yb-doped double tungstates (KYW and KGW) provide a new opportunity for design of practical Yb-based DPSSLs. A continued research is necessary for Yb-based laser crystals amenable to channel waveguide formation and possessing more favorable laser spectroscopic values.

The novel self-frequency doubling Yb:YCOB and Yb:GdCOB crystals seem destined for practical use in visible DPSSL applications. A 10 W Q-switched ultraviolet DPSSL sets a new record in operating at 355 nm.

Diode-pumped solid-state laser sources started replacing gas and ion laser sources for commercial and laboratory applications and the trend is accelerating because of progress in two areas.

First, more powerful, reliable laser diodes are available at lower cost, making diode pumping not only attractive but also practical.

Secondly, advances in manufacturing have improved the quality while reducing the volume pricing for laser crystals such as Nd:YAG and Nd:YVO_4, and nonlinear optical crystals such as β-BaB_2O_4 (BBO), LiB_3O_5 (LBO) and $KTiOPO_4$ (KTP). To meet requirements of expanding laser applications, important progress has occurred in searching out new crystals that can cover broader spectral applications.

2.2.7 Garnets

Some of the most useful laser hosts are the synthetic garnets such as yttrium aluminium garnet or $Y_3Al_5O_{12}$ (YAG), gadolinium gallium garnet or $Gd_3Ga_5O_{12}$ (GGG) and gadolinium scandium gallium garnet or $Gd_3Sc_2Ga_3O_{12}$ (GSGG). These garnets have many desirable properties to use it as laser host material. They are stable, hard, optically isotopic and have good thermal conductivities which permit laser operation at high average power levels. In particular, yttrium aluminium garnet doped with neodymium (Nd:YAG) has achieved a high status among solid-state laser materials. In recent days, ytterbium-doped yttrium aluminium garnet is becoming popular due to the ytterbium's quasi three level. YAG is a very hard, isotropic crystal which can be grown and fabricated in a manner that yields rods of high optical quality. At the present time, it is the best commercially available crystalline laser host for Nd^{3+}, (although several new host materials are available at present) offering low threshold and high gain. The most important ions used in crystal doping for SSLs can be divided into two main classes, viz., transition metal ions and rare earth ions. The most important members of the *transition metal family* are Cr^{3+} and Ti^{3+}. The former was the first to show laser action, using sapphire as host crystal (ruby:Cr^{3+}:Al_2O_3). Titanium used in sapphire shows a very broad tunable emission range which is useful for spectroscopic applications. The *rare earth ions* are the natural candidates to serve as active ions in solid-state laser materials because they exhibit a wealth of sharp fluorescent transitions representing almost every region of the visible and near-infrared portions of the electromagnetic spectrum.

These lines are very sharp, even in the presence of the strong local crystal fields. The other rare earth ions have also shown laser action in many different crystals. Out of several rare earth ions, Nd^{3+} was used as a common dopant for many crystals as well as in glasses. Nd^{3+}, Er^{3+}, Ho^{3+} and Yb^{3+} are becoming popular day-by-day due to their eye safe emission wavelength.

2.2.7.1 *Neodymium* Nd^{3+} was the first trivalent rare earth ions to be used in a laser and it remains as the most important element in this group. Stimulated emission has been obtained with this ion by incorporating it with several host materials. Further, a high power level has been obtained from Nd lasers than from any other four-level material. The principal host materials are YAG and glass. In these hosts, stimulated emission is obtained at a number of frequencies within three different groups of transitions centered at 0.9, 1.06, and 1.35μm

2.2.7.2 *Erbium* Numerous studies of the absorption and fluorescence properties of erbium in various host materials have been conducted to determine its potential as an active laser ion. Laser oscillation was observed most frequently in the wavelength region 1.53 to 1.66 μm. Stimulated emission of around 1.6 μm is of interest to ophthalmologists because the eye is subjected to less retinal damage by laser radiation at 1.6 μm. The reduced transmissivity of the ocular media is the reason for selecting this. The Er:YAG and Er,Cr:YSGG dental lasers are very similar in their basic design and characteristics.

Both laser types use solid-state crystals, YAG or YSGG, doped with erbium ions (Er3+) as their active materials. Also, both lasers are pumped by a pulsed broadband flash lamp.

2.2.7.3 *Holmium* Holmium was discovered by Swedish chemist Per Teodor Cleve (1840-1905) in 1879. Ho is used as a dopant material in glasses or in garnet for producing Ho:YAG or Ho:Glass lasers. It is a rare earth metal and belongs to lanthanide family. Like other rare earth elements, holmium is a silvery metal that is soft, ductile, and malleable. Holmium also has some rather unusual magnetic and electrical properties. Holmium has a melting point of 1,470°C (2,680°F) and a boiling point of 2,720°C (4,930°F). Its density is 8.803 grams per cubic centimeter. Holmium metal tends to be stable at room temperature. In moist air and at higher temperatures, it becomes more reactive. In the past, there were almost no practical uses for holmium and its compounds. However, holmium is now used in specialized lasers. Holmium lasers are used to reduce abnormal eye pressure, to treat glaucoma (an eye disorder), and to repair failed glaucoma surgeries.

2.2.8 Laser Crystals

Among the lot of crystals used as the active media of the solid-state lasers, a few have gained great prominence. The first is ruby (Cr^{3+} in sapphire), both for historical reasons (it was the first laser to be operated) as well as for some unique properties. Next comes the Nd:YAG and all the other Nd-based materials. Recently a new class of materials, viz., Alexandrite and Ti:Sapphire have become popular and they can be used as the tunable laser crystals.

2.2.8.1 *Nd-doped materials* From the large number of Nd-doped materials, only few have prominence. Nd:YAG laser is the most important solid-state laser for scientific, medical, industrial and military applications due to its high gain, good thermal and mechanical properties. Nd:glass is important for laser fusion drivers because it can be produced in large sizes. Very recently, Nd:Cr:GSGG has received considerable attention because of the good spectral match between the flash lamp emission and the absorption of the Cr ions. An efficient energy transfer between the Cr and Nd ions results in a highly efficient Nd laser. Nd:YLF is a good candidate for certain specialized applications because the output is polarized and the crystal exhibits lower thermal birefringence. Nd:YLF has a higher energy storage capability due to its lower gain coefficient compared to Nd:YAG. Further, its output wavelength matches with that of phosphate Nd:glass. Hence mode-locked and Q-switched Nd:YLF lasers have become the standard oscillators for large glass lasers employed in fusion research.

2.2.8.1.1 Nd:YAG The Nd:YAG laser is the most commonly used solid-state laser. Neodymium-doped yttrium aluminium garnet (Nd:YAG) possesses a combination of properties uniquely favorable for laser operation. The YAG host is hard and possesses good optical quality and a high thermal conductivity. Furthermore, the cubic structure of YAG favours a narrow fluorescent line-width which results in high gain and low threshold for laser operation. In Nd:YAG, trivalent neodymium substitutes for trivalent yttrium, so charge compensation is not required. By improving the quality of the material and pumping techniques, CW power can be obtained to several hundred watts from a single laser rod. On the other hand, in single-crystal Nd:YAG fibre lasers, threshold was achieved with absorbed pump powers as small as 1 mW. Today, more than thirty years after its first operation, the Nd:YAG laser has emerged as the most versatile solid-state system. In addition to the very favourable spectral and lasing characteristics displayed by Nd:YAG, the host lattice is noteworthy for its unique physical, chemical, and mechanical properties. The Nd:YAG laser and its energy level diagram are shown in Figures 2.1a and 2.1b, respectively.

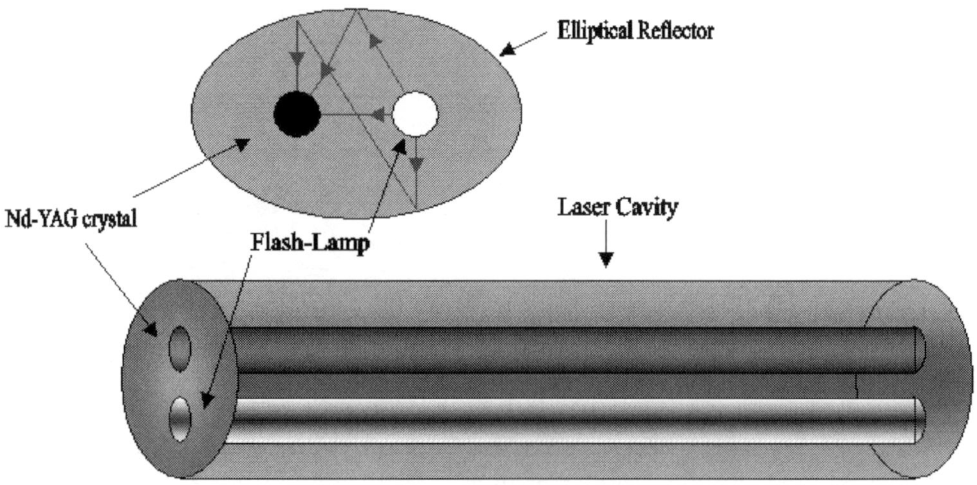

Figure 2.1a Nd:YAG laser (Courtesy: Phy.davidson.edu)

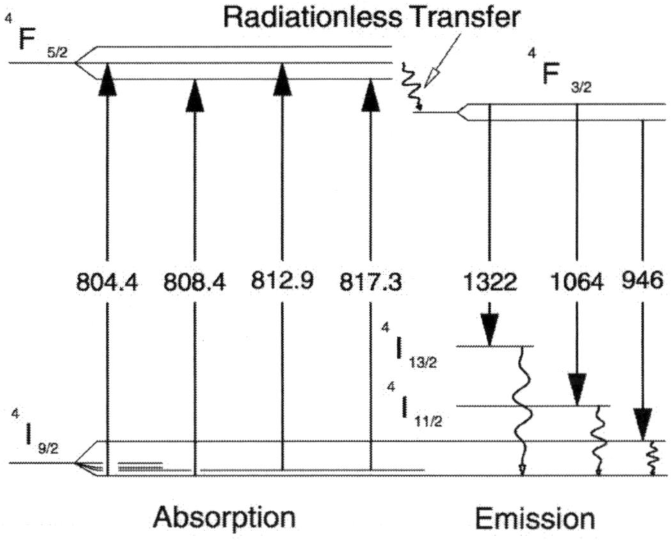

Figure 2.1b Energy level diagram of Nd:YAG (Courtesy: photonics.ld-didactic.com)

The YAG structure is stable from the lowest temperature to the melting point and no transformations have been reported in the solid phase. The strength and hardness of YAG are lower than ruby but still high enough, so that normal fabrication procedures do not produce any serious breakage problems. Pure $Y_3Al_5O_{12}$ is a colorless, optically isotropic crystal which possesses a cubic structure characteristic of garnets. In Nd:YAG, about 1% of Y^{3+} is substituted by Nd^{3+}. The radii of the two rare ions differ by 3%. Therefore, with the addition of large amounts of neodymium, strained crystals are obtained, indicating that either the solubility limit of neodymium is exceeded or that the lattice of YAG is seriously distorted by the inclusion of neodymium.

Commercially available laser crystals are grown exclusively by the Czochralski method. The high manufacturing costs of Nd:YAG are mainly caused by the very slow growth rate of Nd:YAG which is of the order of 0.5 mm/h. Typical boules of 10 to 15 cm in length require a growth run of several weeks. However, all Nd:YAG crystals grown by Czochralski techniques show a bright core running along the length of the crystals. The cores originate from the presence of facets on the growth interface which have a different distribution coefficient for neodymium than the surrounding growth surface. That is, in order to provide rods of a given diameter, the crystal must be grown with a diameter that is somewhat more than twice as large. The boules are processed by quartering into sections. At present times, rods can be fabricated with maximum diameters of about 10 mm and lengths up to 150 mm. The optical quality of such rods is normally quite good and comparable to the best quality of Czochralski ruby or optical glass. For example, 6 mm by 100 mm rods cut from the outer sections of 20 mm by 150 mm boules typically may show only 1 to 2 fringes in a Twyman-Green interferometer.

Neodymium concentration in YAG has been limited to 0.1 to 1.5%. Higher doping levels tend to shorten the fluorescent lifetime, broaden the line-width, and cause strain in the crystal, resulting in poor optical quality. In specifying Nd:YAG rods, the emphasis is on size, dimensional tolerance, doping level, and passive optical tests of rod quality. In a particular application, the performance of a Nd:YAG laser can be somewhat improved by the choice of the optimum Nd concentration. As a general guideline, it can be said that a high doping concentration (approximately 1.2%) is desirable for Q-switch operation because this will lead to high energy storage. For CW operation, a low doping concentration (0.6 to 0.8%) is usually chosen to obtain beam quality. It is worth noting that in contrast to a liquid or a glass, a crystal host is not amenable to uniform dopant concentration. This problem arises as a result of the crystal-growth mechanism. In the substitution of the larger Nd^{3+} for a Y^{3+} in $Y_3Al_5O_{12}$, the neodymium is preferentially retained in the melt. The increase in concentration of Nd from the seed to the final stage of a 20-cm long boule is about 20 to 25%. For a laser rod 3 to 8 cm long, this end-to-end variation may be 0.05 to 0.10% of Nd_2O_3 by weight. The physical and optical properties of Nd:YAG are given in Table 2.3.

Table 2.3 Physical and optical properties of Nd:YAG

Properties	Values
Chemical formula	$Nd:Y_3A_{15}O_{12}$
Crystal structure	Cubic
Lattice constants	12.01
Concentration	~ 1.2 x 1020 cm^{-3}
Melting point	1970°C
Density	4.56 g/cm^3

Mohs hardness	8.5
Refractive index	1.82
Thermal expansion coefficient	7.8 x 10^{-6} /K [111], 0 - 250 °C
Thermal conductivity	14 W/m /K @20 °C, 10.5 W /m /K @100 °C.
Lasing wavelength	1064 nm
Stimulated emission cross section	2.8x10-19 cm^{-2}
Relaxation time of terminal lasing level	30 ns
Radiative lifetime	550 ms
Spontaneous fluorescence	230 ms
Loss coefficient	0.003 cm^{-1} @ 1064 nm
Effective emission cross section	2.8 x 10^{-19} cm^2
Pump wavelength	807.5 nm
Absorption band at pump wavelength	1 nm
Line width	0.6 nm
Polarized emission	Unpolarized
Thermal birefringence	High

2.2.8.1.3 Nd,Cr:GSGG Soon after the invention of the Nd:YAG laser, attempts were made to increase the efficiency of transferring radiation from the pump source to the laser crystal using a second dopant called a "sensitizer". A particularly attractive sensitizer is Cr^{3+} because the broad absorption bands of chromium can efficiently absorb light throughout the whole visible region of the spectrum.

The higher pump efficiency of Nd,Cr:GSGG does not automatically translate into better system performance because Nd,Cr:GSGG does exhibit much stronger thermal focusing and stress birefringence, compared to Nd:YAG. The absorption efficiency and the heat-deposition rate for the Nd,Cr:GSGG rod is almost three times those of Nd:YAG. Hence thermal focusing power as a function of lamp input power is several times larger in Nd,Cr:GSGG than in Nd:YAG. Therefore, if beam brightness is the criteria, rather than output energy, some of the advantage of GSGG is offset, particularly at high-average powers. Tunability of the emission in solid-state lasers is achieved when the stimulated emission of photons is intimately coupled to the emission of vibrational quanta (phonons) in a crystal lattice. In these "vibronic" lasers, the total energy of the lasing transition is fixed but can be partitioned between photons and phonons in a continuous fashion. This results in broad wavelength tunability of the laser output. In other words, the existence of tunable solid-state lasers is due to the subtle interplay between the Coulomb field of the lasing ion, the crystals field of the host lattice, and electron-phonon coupling permitting broadband absorption and emission. Therefore, the gain in vibronic lasers depends on transitions between coupled vibrational and electronic states. That is, a phonon is either emitted or absorbed with each electronic transition. The best known and most used vibronic lasers now available are the Alexandrite and Ti:sapphire lasers.

2.2.9 PUMPING

Many different light sources have been used for the optical excitation of solid-state lasers. They can be divided into two broad classes, viz., the *standard incoherent sources* and the *coherent sources*. The *incoherent sources* are used for pumping until now, because of their lower cost and easy availability. The maximum average power available from lamp-pumped solid-state lasers is also of the order of magnitude higher than that available from laser-pumped systems. This situation is now evolving, because of the recent availability of relatively high-power semiconductors lasers, but their high cost limit the average power level in the watt range. On the other hand, lamp-pumped systems are commercially available in the kW range. The incoherent light sources used for solid-state laser pumping are:

1. *Noble-gas arc and flash lamps* They are the most common sources, and come in many different shapes and technology according to the application of the laser.

2. *Metal vapour arc lamps* They are different from the previous lamps due to the narrow emission spectrum which sometimes leads to a higher efficiency. The main drawbacks of metal vapour arc lamps are the low power capabilities and the CW operation.

3. *Filament lamps* They are made by the same tungsten halogen technology used for illumination and hence they are very cheap and the power supply is very simple. Due to their well-known drawbacks, such as the limited available average power, the low transfer efficiency at CW operation and the broadband blackbody emission spectrum, they are confined to low power and inexpensive Nd:YAG systems.

4. *Sun* There are several examples of solid-state lasers pumped by the solar radiation, using mirrors to collect the light on the crystals. Of course, they depend on the availability of the sources but they are very interesting for space application. In some cases, for example using a Nd,Cr:GSGG crystal, the overall efficiency competes with that of photovoltaic solar cells.

5. *Chemical reactions* They are mainly single-shot devices because the chemicals used for the reaction must be replaced after each shot. The most common of these sources is the flash-bulb similar to that used in old photographic flash-lights.

6. *Light emitting diodes* LEDs are similar to diode lasers in concept but their broader emission bands and especially their wide emission angle give a lower coupling efficiency.

The flash lamps are gas discharge devices generally filled with xenon or krypton gases which give pulsed radiation. But, the arc lamps are basically the same gas discharge devices but designed and optimized to produce continuous radiation. The most common shape of both flash and arc lamps is linear. Other shapes are also available from lamp manufactures. In the early stage of ruby lasers, the helical lamps, U-shaped and point lamps were employed. Linear lamps are now preferred for laser pumping since they are much easier to cool by means of a coaxial water flow confined by a transparent tube. In addition, a cylindrical emitter can be more easily coupled to a laser rod. Since almost 50% of the lamp input power is dissipated as heat, lamp body needs cooling. For small power systems, namely, low energy, low repetition rate pulsed lasers, static or forced gas cooling can be used. For higher power systems, liquid cooling can be used.

Although liquid cooling of flash lamps and D.C krypton arc lamps are occasionally performed using coolants other than water, deionized purified water continues to be the most popular liquid coolant. The purity of the water must be high to prevent the etching of quartz and the attachment of dark deposits to the outside surface of the lamp envelop. In systems where electrical connections and coolant are in contact with one another, the water must be deionized to prevent the shorting or weakening of the starting pulse and to minimize erosion of electrical contacts due to electrolysis. Water resistivity greater than 0.2 megohms is highly recommended. All cooling systems component materials should be plastic, stainless steel, or nickel-plated metal.

The flow velocity of the coolant around the flash lamp must be high in such a way the heat exchange between the lamp walls and the liquid is maximum.

2.2.9.2 PUMPING CAVITIES

Since, lamps and most other incoherent sources, emit light diffusely in any direction, an optical systems is used to collect the light into the laser-active medium. This is usually done with a reflector surrounding the lamp and the laser crystals.

The most widely used pump cavity is a highly reflective elliptical cylinder with the laser rod and pump lamp at each focus. The elliptical configuration is based on the geometrical theorem that rays originating from one focus of an ellipse are reflected into the other focus. Therefore an elliptical configuration transfers energy from a linear source placed at one focus to a linear absorber placed along the second focus. The elliptical configuration is closed by two plane-parallel and highly reflecting end plates. Optically this makes the elliptical cylinder infinitely long.

A single elliptical cylinder can have a cross section with a large or small eccentricity. In one case, the laser rod and lamp are separated by a fairly large distance while in the second case they are close together. If the elliptical cylinder closely surrounds the lamp and rod, then the configuration is known as close-coupled elliptical geometry. This geometry usually results in the most efficient cavity. This cavity has further advantage that it minimizes the weight and size of the laser heads. Such reflectors are made by machining from solid metal blocks usually brass or aluminium. The reflective surface is then optical-grade polished and coated with a suitable reflective film. For Nd:YAG or Nd:glass, the best laser coating is electroplated gold which has a good reflectivity on the main absorption bands of Nd. For crystals requiring blue or ultraviolet pumping (as ruby or Ti:sapphire), vacuum-evaporated aluminum is often used, since it gives higher reflectivity than gold at wavelengths shorter than 500 nm. The other possible technology is to close-coupled, nonfocusing, pump cavity, where the lamp and the rod are placed as close as possible and a reflector closely surrounds them. The various pumping configurations are given in Figure 2.2.

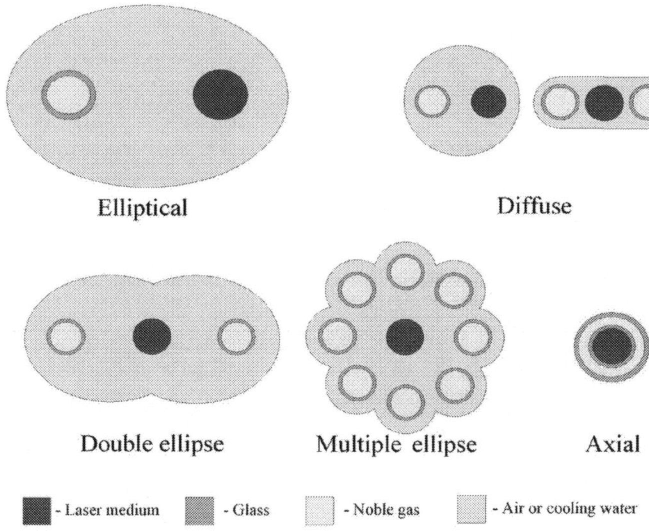

Figure 2.2 Various pumping configurations (Courtesy:commons,Wikimedia.com)

Since all high-average power solid-state lasers are pumped by broadband flash or arc lamps, thermal effects dominate in their operating characteristics. Typically, 5-10% of the power from the exciting flash-lamps is converted to heat within the host material. This heating is due to:

1) energy loss when ions decay from the pump bands to the upper laser level.

2) non-radiative decay of a fraction of the ions in the upper laser level.

3) direct excitation of the host material by the broadband flash-lamp light.

The heat is removed by cooling the laser rod. This leads to the development of a near-parabolic temperature profile in the material. The temperature distribution takes between a few seconds (Nd:YAG) or a minute (Nd:glass) to stabilize. The resulting temperature gradients in an operating laser influence optical behavior. The two mechanisms encountered for this purpose are:

1. They lead to variations in refractive index causing lensing and wavefront distortion, and

2. They produce variations of stress within the body of the material inducing birefringence.

At very high flash-lamp powers, the induced stress can lead to rupture of the laser rod. There are some possible techniques which can be used to compensate for thermal effects in laser rods. Several of these methods can be incorporated within a resonator design. Birefringence problems can be reduced in crystals by selecting the proper orientation of the crystals axes relative to the cylindrical axis. In commercially grown YAG, the rod is along the (111) direction. However, it has been shown that the (001) direction would be preferable for lower losses if the heat dissipation of the rod is lesser than 50W. Generally, losses become independent of orientation axis for powers in excess of 50W. Unfortunately, cutting the (001) direction rod from a (111) grown boule of Nd:YAG limits the size and material waste. Compensation of thermal focussing has been accomplished in many ways, for example, by grinding the ends of the rod to form a negative lens. The cavity mirror selection depends on the negative lens and the rod focal length in the resonator design. It should be noted that each of these passive schemes only provides compensation at one (selected) average pump power. However, many applications require a broad variation of the output power and more complicated adaptive resonator should be used (adaptive mirrors and phase conjugation, etc.).

Since heat is concentrated at the central axis of the cylindrical ruby rod in ruby laser, the material can be removed close to the central axis of the ruby rod. In this way we can remove the heat concentration at the center of the rod. But this gives an annular laser output.

2.2.9.3 SEMICONDUCTOR LASER PUMPING

The most important alternative to flash-lamp pumping of solid-state lasers is the diode laser. In the last twenty-five years, numerous laboratory devices have been assembled which incorporate single diode lasers, small laser-diode arrays or LEDs for pumping of Nd:YAG, Nd:glass and host of other Nd lasers. The low power output, low packaging density and extremely high cost of diode lasers prevented any serious applications for laser pumping in the past. The reason for the continued interest in this area stems from the potential dramatic increase in systems efficiency and component lifetime and reduction of thermal load of the solid-state laser material. The latter will not only reduce thermo-optic effects (which lead to better beam quality) but will also increase pulse repetition frequency. The attractive operating parameters combined with low-voltage operation and the compactness of solid-state laser system have a high potential in applications.

The high pumping efficiency compared to flash lamps stems from the good spectral match between the laser-diode emission and the Nd absorption bands. Actually, flash lamps have higher radiation output to electrical input efficiency (70%) compared to laser diodes (25-50%).

The spectral match between the diode-laser emission and the long-wavelength Nd absorption band reduces the heat deposition in the laser material. Added to this, system lifetime and reliability will be higher in laser-diode-pumped solid-state lasers compared to flash lamp-based systems. Laser-diode arrays have exhibited lifetimes of the order of 19,000 hours in CW operation and 10^9 shots in the pulsed mode. Flash lamp life is of the order of 10^7 shots and about 200 hours for CW operation. In addition, the high pump flux combined with a substantial UV content in lamp-pumped systems cause material degradation in the pump cavity and in the coolant which lead to systems degradation and contribute to maintenance requirements. Such problems are virtually eliminated with laser-diode pump sources. The absence of high-voltage pulses, high temperatures and UV radiation encountered with arc lamps are the special operating features of laser-diode-pumped systems.

In contrast to flash lamps or filament lamps, the emission from laser diode is highly directional and hence require different pump configurations. The techniques for transferring pump radiation from laser diode arrays to the solid-state laser material are discussed below.

We have to distinguish between optical system employed for end-pumping of a laser crystal, side-pumping of a cylindrical rod, and side-pumping of a rectangular slab.

The focused end-pumping configuration is the most efficient pump-radiation transfer scheme, provided the pump light distribution and resonator mode matches (Fig. 2.8). Since, the pump beam from the diode array is collinear with the optical resonator, the overlap between the pumped volume and the TEM_{00} mode can be very high. In addition, the coupling efficiency is high as long as the absorption length is equal to crystal length. In its basic form, end pumping involves a collimating lens with a large numerical aperture in order to collect radiation from a large cone angle and a focusing lens to produce a small diameter spot inside the laser crystal. Since the radiation emitted from a diode array has a high degree of astigmatism, one can introduce prisms or cylindrical optics to transform the beam into a circular shape. The purpose of the coupling optics is to shape the radiation distribution from the diode array such that the pumping volume coincides with the laser's TEM_{00} mode. Radiation from the laser diode array diverges approximately 40 degrees in the plane perpendicular to the active layer. The radiation is collected by a lens. After passing through a pair of prisms, the radiation is focused on the rod by a lens. The resulting divergence inside the Nd:YAG rod is about 6 degrees. In the most common geometry, a plano-concave configuration with high-reflection coating at 1.06 μm at one planar rod surface and anti-reflection coating at 0.81 μm is chosen to allow the pump light to enter the rod. The intra cavity rod surface is anti-reflection-coated at 1.06 μm and an output mirror can be placed either outside the rod or coated directly on the rod itself.

End-pumping of a miniature Nd:YAG laser diode array is an attractive means of obtaining efficient CW lasers. However, at present, the end-pump scheme is useful only for low-power lasers due to the smaller pump area. In order to achieve a somewhat higher output power, two sources can be polarizably coupled to double the pump power or a double-ended pumping arrangement can be employed.

In side-pumping configuration, the diode arrays are placed along the length of the laser rod and pumped perpendicularly to the direction of propagation of the laser. As more power is required, more diode arrays can be added along and around the laser rod. There are three practical approaches to couple the radiation emitted by the diode lasers to the rod.

1. Direct coupling
2. With optics between sources and absorber
3. Fibre-optics coupling

The direct coupling option does not permit for variations other than the position of the diode lasers around the rod. Fibre-optics coupling is very impractical for a large number of diode lasers. Optical coupling can be achieved by using optics such as lenses or elliptical and parabolic mirrors or by non-imaging optics such as reflective or refractive flux concentrators.

The side-pump geometry is not as efficient as the end-pump design. However, it permits scaling of the laser to large power levels. As a matter of fact, the side-pump geometries are normally due to a small absorption length, low pumping density and wasted pump energy due to resonator-mode and pump-distribution mismatch. Large lasers require large rod diameters which increase the pump efficiency. They also require densely packed high-power diode arrays which provide gains over the whole cross section of the rod at sufficient intensity to permit the use of unstable resonators. All these factors contribute to a more efficient utilization of the pump radiation as compared to small systems.

The side-pump geometry is most suitable for slab laser pumping. Side-pumped-slab lasers are usually pumped by 2-D arrays or densely-packed linear arrays. In a slab laser, the face of the crystal and the emitting surface of the laser diodes are in close proximity and no optics is employed. The slab can be pumped from one face only. In this case, the opposite face is bonded to a copper heat sink containing a reflective coating to get back the unused pump radiation to the slab for a second pass. An anti-reflection coating on the pump face is used to reduce coupling losses. Further, liquid cooling is employed to remove heat from the YAG and diode heat sink.

2.3 GAS LASERS

A gas laser consists of a gas or vapour (active medium) whose atoms or molecules are raised to a higher energy state by excitation and hence there exists an inversion between a certain pair of energy levels in the gas. A gas laser essentially consists of 1) a resonator (a long cylindrical glass tube with required gas) 2) an exciting mechanism to cause discharge in the tube and 3) a set of mirrors facing each other. The important types of gas lasers are:

1. Neutral atom lasers (He-Ne laser) and metal vapour (Cu, Au) lasers
2. Molecular gas lasers (CO, CO_2, N_2, CHF_3 lasers)
3. Ion lasers (Ar, Kr, He-Cd lasers)
4. Excimer lasers (rare earth halide lasers, KrF, XeCl)

Gas lasers can be fabricated in many sizes and configurations. The optical, thin film, vacuum, instrument and electrical technologies are involved in the construction of gas lasers. The four main essential parts of gas lasers are the following:

1. Plasma tube and cathodes,
2. Optical components, Brewster windows and dielectric coated mirrors
3. Mechanical mounts and fixtures, etc.
4. Electrical power supply

In addition to the above, vacuum is a very important parameter in gas lasers. This process is essential to remove absorbed gas molecules from the plasma tubes before filling with noble gases or mixtures. The ordinary gas lasers vary in length from 30 to 100 cm. The gas leakage occurs from the walls of the glass tube due to the collision of active gas molecules with the walls. Hence it is impossible to obtain the laser output proportional to the cross sectional area of the tube.

The gas lasers are usually electrically excited by gas discharge using direct current, radio frequency or pulse source. In a few cases, gas dynamic expansion and chemical pumping are also used as excitation mechanisms. The gas lasers are also excited through optical pumping by means of another laser.

The electrical discharge in gas lasers falls under two categories. The first category is due to the excitation by electron impact and can be represented as

$$e + X \rightarrow X + e$$

This is known as collision of the first kind. The second category is due to the excitation by resonant energy transfer and it can be represented as

$$A + B \rightarrow A + B + DE \quad (DE < kT)$$

This is known as collision of second kind.

The collision of second kind, the collision between atoms and molecules, collision with walls of container and stimulated and spontaneous emission causes de-excitation of excited levels.

A population inversion between two given levels will occur when the excitation rate R is greater for upper laser level than for lower laser level.

2.3.1 MOLECULAR GAS LASERS

Molecular lasers take the advantage of transition between energy levels of a molecule. Based on the laser transition, we have three different categories of lasers.

1) *Vibronic lasers* In vibronic lasers (a contraction from the words vibrational and electronic), transition occurs between vibrational levels belonging to different electronic states. In this case, emission wavelengths fall from the UV to the visible region.

2) *Vibrational-rotational lasers* In vibrational-rotational lasers, transition occurs between different vibrational and rotational levels of the electronic ground state. These lasers emit radiation in the mid-IR to far infrared (5-300 μm). For example, CO_2 laser ($\lambda = 9$ to 11 μm) and CO_2 laser ($\lambda = 5$ to 6 μm).

3) *Pure rotational lasers* In rotational laser, transition occurs between different rotational levels within a vibrational state of the electronic ground state. The corresponding emission wavelength is in the far-IR region (25 μm to 1 mm). For example, CH_3F laser ($\lambda = 496$ μm). These lasers are usually optical pumped with CO_2 lasers.

Among the various gas lasers, we will concentrate only on carbon dioxide lasers. Carbon dioxide lasers are the widely used molecular gas lasers for several applications in industry and medicine. It is based on vibrational transitions of carbon dioxide molecule. Hence to understand the working of a molecular laser, one has to know the vibrational modes of the concerned molecule. The fundamental modes of vibration of a CO_2 molecule are illustrated in Figure 2.3.

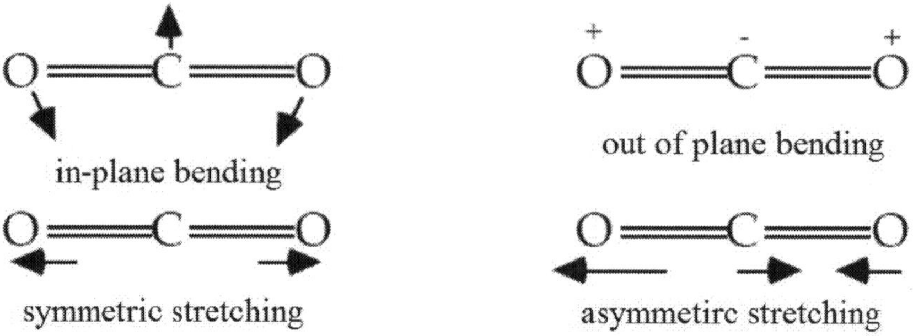

Figure 2.3 Vibrational modes of a carbon dioxide molecule (Courtesy: Skepticalscience.com)

Carbon dioxide molecule possesses three different independent modes. They are symmetric stretching mode n_1 (1,0,0), bending mode n_2 (0,1,0) and asymmetric stretching mode n_3 (0,0,1). The simplified energy levels of all three modes in a single energy level diagram are shown in Figure 2.4. Only the four lowest excited levels are shown in the figure because they are the only ones that take part in the lasing. The energy state of the molecule is represented by the three numbers (*i, j, k*) which represents the amount of energy or number of energy quanta, associated with each mode. The upper laser level is state (001), the lower laser level is provided by state (020) and (100). The transition (001) → (100) yields a line at the wavelength $\lambda = 10.6\ \mu$m whereas the (001) → (020) gives a line at 9.6 μm. States (020) and (100) decay into the ground state mainly by resonant energy transfer to the unexcited CO_2 molecules so that these accumulate in the (010) state. The depopulation of state (010) is the bottleneck of the process. To overcome this, special additives such as helium or water vapour are introduced in the gas mixture. Hence the level degrades due to the collisions with additives.

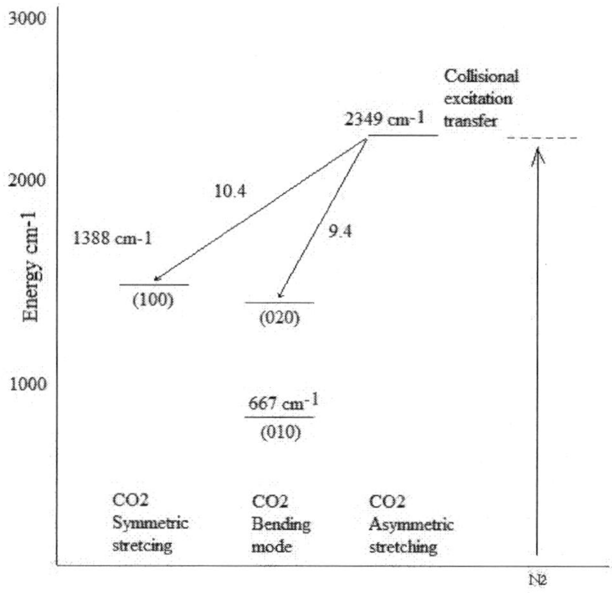

Figure 2.4 Vibrational energy levels of carbon dioxide (Courtesy: Phy.davidson.edu)

All commercial CO_2 lasers are based on vibrational transition within the ground electronic state process. Most CO_2 lasers require a mixture of three gases, viz., carbon dioxide, molecular nitrogen and diverse additives such as helium. The nitrogen gas provides collisional excitation for the carbon dioxide while helium has high thermal conductivity. This property helps to keep the gases cool. The helium efficiently transports heat to the outside of the laser. The nitrogen in the CO_2 discharge takes the role that helium plays in the helium-neon laser.

Carbon dioxide lasers are commercially important because they can generate very high powers with relatively high electrical efficiency. The lasers with average power greater than 20 kW are available and the kilowatt CO_2 lasers are common. The powerful lasers are line tunable and emit radiation in the mid-IR region. They find an extensive application in incisional and excisional biopsies, frenectomy, gingivectomy, pre-prosthetic procedures, soft tissues, dentin desensitization.

The operation characteristics of a CO_2 laser are given in Table 2.4.

Table 2.4 The operation characteristics of a CO_2 laser

Parameters	Values
Gas pressure	Mbar (longitudinal discharge) 100 mbar (wave guide lasers) > 1 bar (TEA laser)
Gas mixture	CO_2:N_2:He 1:1:8
Gas discharge	DC, rf, pulsed, TEA
Laser power	Watts to >20 kilowatts. Continuous wave - kW to TW pulsed.
Total efficiency	Greater than 10%

A typical data of CO_2 laser types are given below.

In general, there are 5 major types of CO_2 lasers. They are:

1) Sealed or no-flow,
2) Slow axial flow,
3) Fast axial flow,
4) Fast transverse flow, and
5) Transverse excited atmosphere (TEA).

2.4 SEMICONDUCTOR LASERS

At present, nearly 80% of the entire laser market is dominated by semiconductor lasers or laser arrays which are used to pump other solid-state lasers or operate with a coherent output from a two-dimensional array. Output powers in excess of one kilowatt with more than 10 per cent power efficiency should become commercially available. These lasers will provide a major boost for industrial processing and medical applications.

Monolithic diode lasers which operate without an external cavity have spectral linewidths that are typically, 30 MHz at output power levels of about 10mW. Such spectral linewidths are not useful for a wide range of applications such as radar, optical heterodyne communications and high resolution spectroscopy.

The source of the spectral broadening in these semiconductor diode lasers is fundamental and quantum in nature and arises from the spontaneous emission noise within the laser. This spontaneous emission noise causes the phase of the electric field vector of the radiation to fluctuate which in turn leads to a spectral broadening. In addition, damped relaxation oscillators due to the perturbation of the field amplitude by spontaneous emission give rise to side bands. These side bands are typically 1–2 GHz away from the main peak. When such devices are placed into high Q external cavities, the linewidths are significantly reduced. The linewidths of less than 400 Hz have been produced in such lasers. The frequency stability characteristics of free-running external-cavity GaAlAs diode lasers which have already been demonstrated are listed in Table 2.5.

Table 2.5 The frequency stability characteristics of free-running external-cavity GaAlAs diode lasers

Property	**Values**
Fundamental width	<1000 Hz
Future capability	<10 MHz
Short-term jitter	5 kHz/30 ms
Long-term jitter	7 kHz
Centre frequency drift	5 kHz/h
Locking stability	<10 mHz
Baseband noise	+/- 0.5GHz +/-0.5 GHz <100 dB

Extending the useful frequency range of presently available diode lasers such as GaAlAs can be accomplished by the use of efficient nonlinear frequency conversion. Wide band gap semiconductor diode lasers have been very difficult to operate at wavelengths shorter than 600 nm. The materials of choice would be the II-VI compounds but so far have not proven to operate as diodes because of the inability to fabricate *p*-type material. Therefore, nonlinear frequency conversion would be one solution for the near-term operation of compact blue diode laser sources.

The blue laser is a laser that emits electromagnetic radiation at a wavelength of between 360 and 480 nm, which the human eye sees as blue light or else light at the blue end of the spectrum. Diode lasers which emit light at 445 nm are becoming popular as laser pointers. Lasers emitting wavelengths below 445 nm appear violet to the human eye, a distinctly different color. This is true, for example, of the most commercially common "blue" lasers, the diode lasers used in Blue-ray applications, which emit 405 nm light that is violet. This light causes fluorescence in some chemicals, in the same way that ultraviolet or "black light" does. The class of blue lasers are frequently semiconductor laser diodes based on gallium (III) nitride (violet color) or indium gallium nitride (often true-blue in color, but able to produce other colors, as well). Both blue and violet lasers can also be constructed using frequency-doubling of infrared laser wavelengths from diode lasers or diode-pumped lasers. Devices that employ blue laser light have applications in many areas ranging from optoelectronic data storage at high density to medical applications.

Major advances in high-power diode lasers have been made in the world with the development of the graded index separate confinement heterostructure GaAlAs diode laser. These lasers have produced over one watt of CW power at room temperature with more than 50% power conversion efficiency. One problem with these monolithic devices is the poor spectral output. This may be improved by operation in an external cavity. Because the broadening mechanism in semiconductor lasers leads to a homogeneous gain line, all of the laser output will occur in a single frequency when the devices are operated in a single spatial mode. Such a diode laser has been operated in an external cavity and has produced more than 1.5 watts of continuous power at room temperature in a spectral width of less than 8 GHz and a spatial beam quality which was better than 2-3 times diffraction limited. Because of the energy band properties of quantum-well laser materials, the gain bandwidths can be very broad. A single such laser when operated in an external cavity with a grating has been continuously tuned from 790 to 860 nm at room temperature. Two such lasers have covered the range from 720 to 870 nm. Frequency-doubling of such high-power devices would produce useful radiation from 360 to 435 nm with additional tuning over the entire visible range possible by parametric conversion.

The use of efficient diode lasers and diode laser arrays are now in widespread use as efficient pump sources for solid-state lasers to provide all solid state, compact, reliable and efficient lasers which are able to produce output from a few mW to 100 W. Such lasers would find numerous applications where the disadvantages of lamp pumping are obvious. The most common material that has been pumped by diode lasers is Nd:YAG which has its main output lines at 1.06 and 1.32 μm.

Table 2.6 Properties and Applications of Semiconductor lasers

Laser gain medium and type	Operation wavelength(s)	Pump source	Applications
Semiconductor laser diode	Wavelength depends on device material: 0.4 μm, (GaN) or 0.63 μm–1.55 μm (AlGaAs) or 3–20 μm (lead salt)	Electrical current	Telecommunications, holography, laser pointers, printing, pump sources for other lasers. The 780 nm AlGaAs laser diode, used in compact disc players, is the most common type of laser in the world.

2.6 FIBRE LASERS

Fibre lasers are particularly efficient at converting the often poor beam quality obtained from a diode laser into diffraction-limited laser radiation. In a fibre laser, the active ion is doped into the central core of an optical fibre, the ions being pumped by radiation propagating along the fibre axis. Fibre lasers have several advantages over the traditional rod or disc geometries.

1) *Low pump power threshold* Achievement of the threshold population inversion density requires the pump laser to exceed a threshold intensity. Since the cross-sectional area of an optical fibre is so low, the power required to reach threshold is orders of magnitude smaller than in a rod or disc where the area of the gain medium is at least an order of magnitude larger. In practice threshold pump powers significantly below 1 mW can be achieved. Using the fibre laser geometry it is possible to achieve lasing in lasers with low gain coefficients; with high threshold pump intensities; and even in three-level laser systems.

2) *Guiding of pump beam* The pump laser radiation is naturally guided by the fibre, allowing very long gain regions to be employed.

3) *High efficiency* The good overlap between the pump and generated laser radiation along the whole length allows efficient conversion of the pump laser energy into laser output.

4) *Good thermal management* For any solid-state laser system it is important to conduct away pump energy deposited into the gain medium in the form of heat, in order to avoid thermal lensing. The high surface area to volume ratio of the fibre geometry allows heat to be conducted away more effectively.

5) *Compact gain medium* Optical fibres may be coiled, keeping the volume of the laser system small.

6) *Robustness* Optical fibres are robust and much less liable to cracking or other physical damage.

The main disadvantages of fibre lasers are that the volume of the gain region is small. Consequently the energy stored in the gain region will also be small, and hence fibre lasers are not useful for amplifying laser pulses to high energy. Further, the long propagation length through the fibre core can be associated with the development of non-linear loss processes such as stimulated Raman scattering or stimulated Brillouin scattering.

2.6.1 Erbium-doped fibre lasers

Silica optical fibres have transmission windows at 1.3 μm and 1.5 μm. Single-mode fibres used at 1.3 μm have low dispersion and so the distance that signals can propagate before they must be amplified or regenerated is determined primarily by the fibre loss of 0.4 $dBkm^{-1}$. Amplifiers are not available at 1.3 μm, and so signals at this wavelength are regenerated in a regenerative repeater, which: (i) detects and interprets the signal; (ii) corrects errors; and (iii) regenerates and retransmits the bit stream. The optimum repeater separation is typically 40 km.

Amplification can be provided by an erbium-doped fibre amplifier (EDFA). The EDFA operates on the $^4I_{13/2} \rightarrow {}^4I_{15/2}$ transition at approximately 1550 nm. As discussed previously, pump radiation can conveniently be provided by diode lasers operating at 800, 980, or 1480 nm.

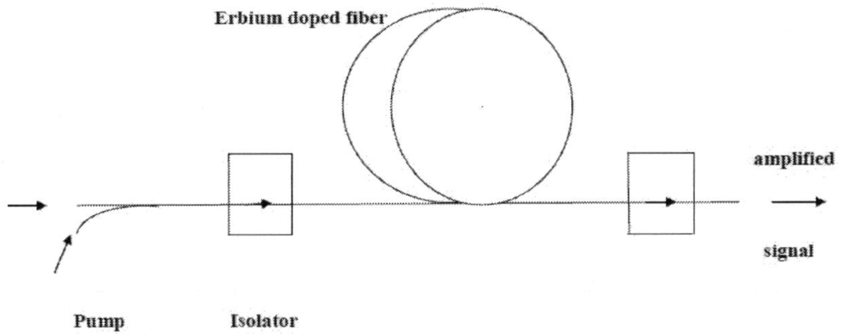

Figure 2.5 Schematic diagram of an EDFA

Figure 2.5 shows schematically the configuration of an EDFA. The pump laser radiation is coupled into the amplifier by splicing together a fibre carrying the pump radiation and a fibre coaxial with the amplifier. The amplifying section is a monomode silica fibre doped with around 0.1% erbium, and with a length ranging from metres to hundreds of metres. The single-pass gain is typically of order 10^3. Notice that optical isolators based on the Faraday effect are inserted around the EDFA to prevent parasitic laser oscillation arising from the small Fresnel reflections at junctions in the fibre. EDFAs have been used in the latest 5 $Gbit.s^{-1}$ transatlantic fibres which employ amplifiers every 35 km, but only regenerate the signal at the two land stations!

Finally we note that the very wide bandwidth (some 30 nm or 3.74 THz) of the erbium transition allows amplification of multiple channels each transmitted at a slightly different wavelength. This technique, wavelength division multiplexing (WDM), could allow, for example, 375 channels of 2.5 $Gbit.s^{-1}$ and spaced by 10 GHz to be transmitted within the bandwidth of an erbium amplifier. The implementation of WDM, however, requires the development of suitable laser sources and techniques for de-multiplexing the transmitted signals; a great deal of work is being done in this area.

References

[1] A.A. Kaminskii. 1996. *"Crystaline Lasers: Physical Processes and Operating Schemes"*, CRC Press, Section 1.4.5, ISBN:0-8493-3720-8.

[2] Early work on diode pumping of Ho:YAG can be found in: T.Y. Fan, et al., *Opt. Lett.*, 12, 678 (1987) along with R. Allen et al., *Electron. Lett.*, 22, 947 (1986).

[3] S. Lamrini, et al. 2010. "High-Power Ho:YAG Laser in-Band Pumped by Laser Diodes at 1.9 μm and wavelength-stabilized by a Volume Bragg Grating" ASSP 2010 *Technical Digest*, ISBN 978-1-55752-883-4.

[4] Xiaodong Mu, et al. 2010. "High Efficiency, High Power 2.097-μm Ho:YAG Laser", ASSP 2010 *Technical Digest*, ISBN 978-1-55752-883-4.

[5] A. Einstein. 1916. "Zur Quantum Theorie Der Stralung" *Verk Deutch Phys*. Ges. 18 (1916) 318.

[6] T.H. Maiman. 1960. "Stimulated optical radiation in ruby", *Nature* 187 (1960) 493-494.

[7] Leo J. Miserendino. 1995. History and development of Laser Dentistry: in *Lasers in Dentistry*, Leo J. Miserendino, Robert M. Pick, Quintessence Publishing Co. Inc., Singapore, p. 17.

3

Laser Light-Tissue Interactions

Dr. V. Arjunan

Head of the Department of Chemistry,

Arignar Anna Government ,

Arts & Scence College, Karaikal - 609 605

Dr. Sujin P.Jose

School of Physics,

Madurai Kamaraj University,

Madurai 625 021, India

3.1 INTRODUCTION

Understanding lasers begins with understanding the acronym LASER—light amplification by the stimulated emission of radiation. All states of matter—solids, liquids and gases—contain potential energy and can be stimulated to emit it in packets of light called photons. When a stimulated atom absorbs a photon, energy states of electron changes causing the emission of a series of identical photons. Argon gas, CO_2 gas, ruby crystals, Nd:YAG crystals, liquid dyes and other mediums are capable of absorbing the emitting photons of various wavelengths. Long-wavelength photons with low levels of energy and short wavelength photons with high intensity have different biological effects in tissue. The difference in tissue effects on lasers depend on their degree of absorption in target tissue and energy delivery scheme. Ultimately thermal effects of the laser play an important role in precise surgical effects.

Laser wavelengths are found not only in the visible range but also in the infra-red and ultraviolet region of the electromagnetic spectrum and they are non-ionizing radiations. That is, laser light does not accumulate in cells and cannot cause cellular change or damage as X-rays and gamma radiation.

Laser light is different from ambient light because it is coherent, collimated and monochromatic. These unique properties make lasers to work as surgical tools. The coherent property of laser light uniformly absorbs energy, with minimal loss of energy. Coherence helps to focus a beam sharply by an optical system. Precise collimation reduces the diffusion of energy and allows delivery as an intense beam through mirrors or fibre optics. This concentrated energy does not disperse in space and produces a beam that holds its intensity until it is bent, absorbed or changed mechanically. Laser light is monochromatic—all in one colour or wavelength. It is this property that enables us to use the light to surgically alter tissue.

The effects of the laser beam on the biological tissues are as follows:

1) Thermal effects are produced by most continuous wave lasers such as CO_2, YAG and argon. The laser energy is absorbed by the biological tissue, raising the local temperature, so the tissue can be ablated, vaporized, coagulated or cut.

2) Mechanical effects arise especially when short pulses of high power laser is used to create a "blast" by heating a small region of tissue to high temperature in a very short time. The blast creates a shock wave that disrupts the tissue nearby. This effect is used in eye treatment for disrupting posterior capsule in secondary cataract.

3) Chemical effects are used in photo-dynamic therapy (PDT). Excimer lasers are employed in reshaping the cornea.

4) Optical Processes—The parameter that summarizes the effects of laser radiation on biological tissue is fluence.

$$\text{Fluence} = (\text{Watt X time})/\text{Spot size}$$

When a laser beam falls on matter, four processes can take place. They are 1) reflection, 2) scattering, 3) transmission, and 4) absorption. Only absorption can transfer energy to the material so that there is a rise in temperature or chemical reaction.

The interaction between electromagnetic radiation and biological tissue depends on:

1. The wavelength of light which determines the energy of each photon of light.

2. The intensity of radiation.

3. The shape of irradiation (continuous or pulsed).

For power levels up to few watts, the interaction is divided into 3 regions of wavelengths.

1. Short UV region—the photons interact with the proteins, RNA and DNA and usually kill the biological cells.

2. Near-UV and short visible range—cause photochemical reactions such as photosynthesis, especially with the Excimer laser.

3. Visible and near infrared region—thermal effects due to absorption of the radiation.

When using lasers for medical treatments, a good understanding of the interaction between specific laser radiation with specific biological tissue is required.

Each wavelength interacts differently with body tissue and each creates different types of surgical or medical effects. Hence, many types of medical lasers such as carbon dioxide, Nd:YAG, Ho:YAG, argon, KTP, dye, alexandrite, ruby and diode are available and no one system can perform all types of procedures. Further the type of emission whether it is continuous or pulsed is also an important factor as far as medical application is concerned. The duration of the emission can vary according to the excitation duration from milliseconds to nanoseconds. The energy and the power densities are usually important. The small focal spot in which the beam is concentrated by a proper laser can reach up to hundreds of J/cm to MW/cm.

Laser light has four main characteristics that determine how each wavelength can be used in tissues. The tissue–radiation interactions are transmission, absorption, scattering, and reflection. Each of these properties affects the laser cutting, coagulation or vaporization of tissues. A through understanding of these four characteristics of light with tissues is necessary before the physician selects the correct laser system for a particular application.

Absorption is the way a laser interacts with biological material in tissue. The main substances that absorb light are water, protein, melanin, and haemoglobin. The carbon dioxide laser is a multipurpose laser because it is absorbed by water. Since most body cells are composed with more than 85% water, the light is easily absorbed. Light radiations develop heat when absorbed by the tissues and hence the intracellular water begins to boil. They swell continuously until they disrupt by emitting water vapour, carbon, and cellular particulates. Vaporization of cells allows for precise, rapid removal of tissue, as well as excellent excision, incision, and dissection. CO_2 laser does not coagulate well due to its affinity for water and will seal only the smallest vessels under 0.5 mm in diameter.

Nd:YAG (neodymium, yttrium, ytterbium and garnet crystal) laser, not only passes through water but is also absorbed in tissue protein, coagulating up to 6 mm. It is the most haemostatic of all surgical lasers with the ability to seal a bleeding vessel of up to 1.5 mm. Since CO_2 laser travels so deeply into tissue, it does not cut or vaporize and can damage peripheral tissues if not carefully controlled. The CO_2 (10,600 nm) and the Nd:YAG (1064 nm) are invisible and hence they require an auxiliary low-power, visible, aiming laser beam. Most lasers use a helium–neon (630 nm) laser of very low intensity as an aiming beam. Interestingly, this aiming beam has no independent effect on tissue.

Depending on the temperature, many kinds of changes can occur in the biological system. As tissue begins to heat above 60°C, it begins to desiccate, blanch white and shrink as proteins denature and flash boil at 100°C. Different lasers cause absorptive heating as follows:

Temp in °C	**Visual change**	**Biological change**
100+	Smoke plume	Vaporisation, carbonisation
90–100	Pluckering	Drying, elimination of fluids

65–90	White/grey	Protein denaturation
60–65	Blanching	Coagulation
37–60	None	Warming, welding

Visible wavelengths (Argon, KTP, dyes) are absorbed by chromophores in tissues of opposite colour. The blue-green argon (488, 514 nm) is highly absorbed in red-brown structures that contain melanin and/or haemoglobin. Argon transmits through water and is shallow in its penetration (2–3 nm) so that it can be used to coagulate superficial vessels with precision and safety.

KTP works by changing the frequency of Nd:YAG (1064 nm) by passing it through a crystal of potassium titanyl phosphate (KTP) which doubles the frequency and results in a visible green beam (532 nm). KTP works very much like argon in absorption mechanism and tissue effects. It can be delivered through fibres and transmits easily through water and is an effective endoscopic tool.

Other visible wavelengths, such as dye lasers (575–850 nm) are more useful on light brown and pink lesions. Visible light lasers are the most effective for ophthalmic surgery and for both vascular and pigmented dermatologic lesions. A large number of these lasers are available in the market with both Q-switching and pulsed mechanisms and delivery by both articulated arms or fibre optics.

In order to work as a surgical tool, laser light must be transmitted into the tissue. Lasers are very different from electrical energy in their effects on tissue. Electrical energy travels along the path of least resistance, causing uncontrollable areas of injury. Its depth of penetration and lateral zone of destruction cannot be predetermined. It cannot produce the precise effects of laser energy which is absorbed by tissue components such as water, protein and pigment.

Laser action can be achieved in almost every material within the proper operating condition. The active medium can be solid, liquid or gaseous phase. The transition can be rotational, vibrational, electronic, atomic or molecular for the different laser wavelengths. All of them possess the fundamental property such as monochromaticity, directionality, spatial and temporal coherence.

For CW lasers the power of the radiation defines completely the energy content. For pulsed lasers, pulse duration is usually defined at full width half maximum

(FWHM). The repetition rate of the pulses determines the average power as the product of the single pulse energy times and the repetition rate.

The relevance of laser parameters in dental applications is given in Table 3.1

Table 3.1 Relevance of laser parameters in dental applications

Parameter	Relevance	Effects
Brightness	Very high	Intense local heating, non-contact interaction
Spatial coherence	Moderate	Extreme focusability, optical fibre coupling
Pulsed power	Moderate	Continued thermal effects, nonlinear processes
Tunability	Moderate	Selective absorption, (chromophores, sensitizers)
Monochromaticity	Low	Extreme focusability

The effects of laser on tissues can be listed as:

1) Tissue heating: a) Skin rejuvenation, b) Tissue welding

2) Coagulation: a) Haemostasis, b) Protein with attendant necrosis

3) Vaporisation: a) Cutting (ablating along a fine line with traction),

   b) Debulking (ablating volumes of tissues)

4) Non-linear effects: a) Cold cutting–ophthalmic Nd:YAG,

   b) Photoacoustical "Lithotripsy"

   c) Fragmentation of tattoo pigment via, Q-switched lasers (Here the shock waves rip and tear the tissues. In ophthalmic case, it creates tiny sparks in thin air which tear apart the clouded membrane behind the lens.)

5) Photochemistry: a) Photodynamic therapy (PDT)

6) Photodissociation: a) Non-thermal ablation of the cornea in ophthalmology (This is vision correction laser. The laser wavelength of 193 nm removes tissue without heat generation).

In general, laser is actually vaporizing the cells when they cut or debulk tissues. Further, the way the energy is delivered in terms of its peak power, pulse duration and spot size are more important than the wavelength in the clinical choice of laser system. The tissue reaction with lasers is shown in Figure 3.1.

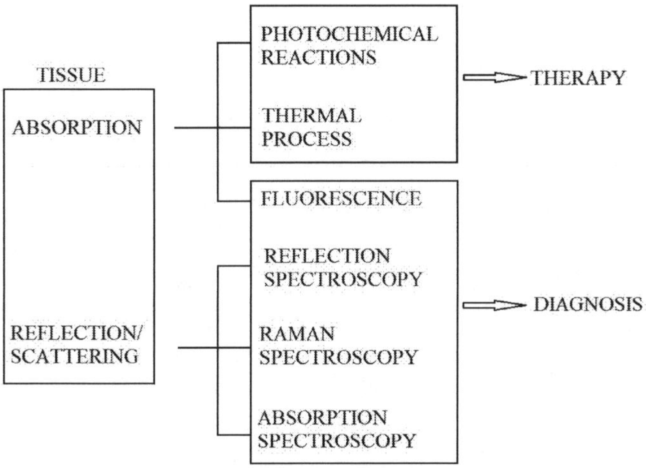

Figure 3.1 Tissue reaction with laser

3.2 PHOTOPHYSICAL PROCESS IN LASER-TISSUE INTERACTIONS

A good amount of research has been done on the photobiological interaction between non-ionising radiation and living tissues in the submillimeter part of electromagnetic spectrum and in the optical region. In the specific case of laser radiation, the unique characteristic of monochromaticity of the incident field and the spatial and temporal coherence of the emission, find increasing use in medical applications, in both diagnosis and therapy. The primary interaction of laser light with tissue is shown in Figure 3.2.

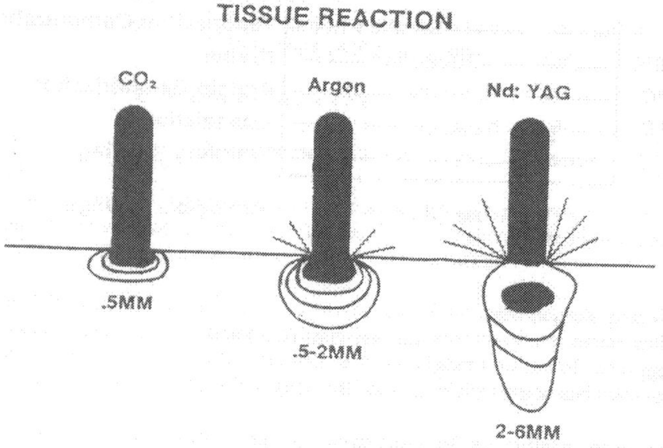

Figure 3.2 Laser–tissue interaction (Courtesy:industriallaser.com)

The biological response of the irradiated tissue is due to the various processes of conversion of the incident electromagnetic energy within biomolecules. Figure 3.3 shows a plot of power density and interaction time for different effects.

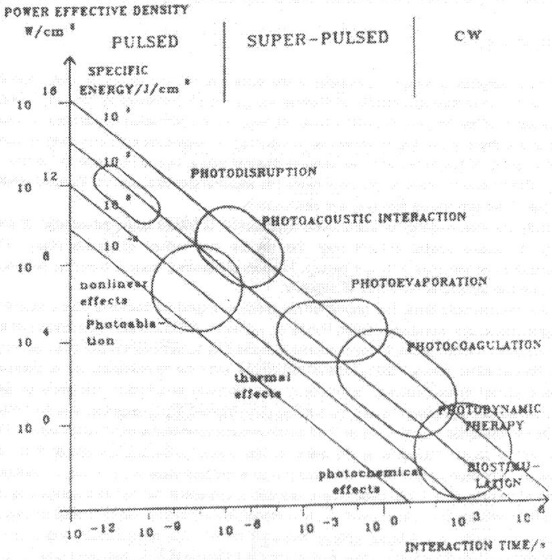

Figure 3.3 Laser-tissue interactions as a function of interaction time and power density (Courtesy: Lasers Med Sci. 1986, 1:47–66)

The specific modes of interaction of laser radiation with tissue, characterises the various applications in diagnosis and therapy. The effect of laser radiation on body tissue depends on the 1) absorption characteristics of the tissue, 2) the characteristics of the laser radiation and 3) on biological effects consequent to the interaction. A detailed understanding has not yet been developed, although the details about interactions are well-known. The most dominant mechanisms are a thermal process following absorption of the laser radiation. The mid-infrared 10.6 μm beam of the CO_2 laser is strongly absorbed by the high water content in cellular tissue. The water is heated and vapourized tissue disrupts. This is characterised by an interaction distance of less than 1 mm for the CO_2 laser and typically 6 mm for the tunable dye (0.340–1.1 μm), Nd:YAG (1.06 μm) and Argon (0.485–0.515 μm). The intermediate absorption distance of laser radiation by tissues causes volume interaction with scattering and weak absorption. But the strong absorption distance causes surface interaction with low scattering of radiation. The wavelength, nature of absorption and nature of interaction of four commonly used lasers are given below.

Laser	**Tunable Dye**	**Nd:YAG**	**CO_2**	**Argon**
Wavelength	0.340–1.1 μm	1.06 μm	10.6 μm	0.485–0.515 μm
Nature of absorption	Intermediat absorption	Weak absorption	Strong absorption	Scattering
Nature of interaction	Volume interaction	Volume interaction	Surface interaction	Low scattering

The absorption by water at the Nd:YAG laser wavelength is low and the beam is mainly absorbed by haemoglobin and pigmented tissue. Hence, it has an intermediate characteristic absorption distance. With absorption of the laser radiation, the tissue cells are destroyed and it is often important to minimize damage to surrounding normal tissue. When this is well vascularised, such as in the gastrointestinal tract or in the liver, damage to adjacent tissue is limited to about 0.1 mm for the CO_2 laser, about 1 mm for the argon laser and approximately 6 mm for the Nd:YAG laser. It is seen that the effect of the CO_2 laser is highly localised and this leads to the use of the laser for surgical cutting. The interaction volume with argon laser is grater and with the Nd:YAG, it is still great. Scattering in the inhomogeneous tissue with the Nd:YAG laser leads to a volume of interaction several times larger than the laser spot size.

The thermal contraction which occurs initially causes sealing of small blood vessels and coagulation with a reduction in haemorrhage. Coagulation with CO_2 laser is mainly by conduction from the laser beam and the largest size of blood vessel which can be sealed is limited to about 1 mm. The larger interaction volume of the Nd:YAG laser enables larger vessels to be sealed. The advantages of good excision with the CO_2 laser and coagulation with the Nd:YAG laser can be best achieved by incorporating both lasers in a new laser arrangement.

When power levels are insufficient to produce substantial heating, biophysical effects may occur by biostimulation or through the use of tissue sensitising agents. Although the biostimulation mechanism is uncertain, one possible mechanism for low levels of laser radiation is to stimulate cell division so that the rate of biological process is increased (For example, in the rate of healing of skin ulcers). This area is presently being further explored with argon and He-Ne lasers.

By various mechanisms, high power pulsed laser interacts with tissues. The output of pulsed laser can be of duration 10^{-3}, 10^{-6} or 10^{-8} seconds or even shorter. The instantaneous high power of the laser beam when focussed on the tissue produces sufficiently high electrical fields for electrical breakdown and sufficiently high temperature to form a plasma, causing disruption of the surface. Excimer lasers produce ultraviolet radiation in the range 193-315 nm which is strongly absorbed by biological tissues and with a 10^{-7} second laser pulse, the surface can be photo-ablated. Since the focal spot size of the excimer laser is a few microns, a very small and well defined region can be selectively destroyed. There are five basic types of laser–tissue interaction. They are:

1. Photothermal

Laser light (above intensity threshold) falling on tissue produces heat and hence there is a rise in temperature. The radiations are absorbed by water, tissue pigments and proteins. Such absorption is wavelength-dependent.

2. Photodisruptive

The pulsed laser energy associated with acoustic energy (Photoacoustic high-pressure acoustic wave) causes mechanical interaction with the tissue. This type of photomechanical interaction is dependent on peak power and not on wavelength.

3a. Photochemical

Laser radiations (low intensity and wavelength-selective) are used for photo-excitation and hence the chemical energy breaks the chemical bonds or excite the molecules to reactive state. The short wavelengths are used for photochemical interactions.

3b. Photodynamic (Photochemical and photoablation)

Photodynamic interaction activates singlet oxygen from specific molecules. The specific wavelengths are employed for photoablation.

4. Bio-stimulation

Low power laser radiation is used for healing skin ulcers. Research is on the way in this area and the laser healing mechanism will be clear in future.

5. Photomechanical

This term usually defines mechanical interaction of the target with the acoustic wave associated to the transient absorption of a pulsed radiation. It is used in laser lithotripsy.

3.2.1 Photothermal Interactions

All laser surgical applications, whether in the cutting or haemostatic mode, rely upon the conversion of electromagnetic energy to thermal energy. This is achieved by focusing a beam onto spot sizes of few micrometers or millimeters wide. Such collimation is possible because of the spatial coherence of lasers which can supply high energy densities. The spatially confined heating of target tissue helps in tissue removal, control of bleeding and in thermal injury. The choice of wavelength determines the depth of penetration and thus influences the interplay between tissue removal and haemostasis.

In fact, the vast majority of therapeutic application of lasers takes advantages of their capability for some spatial control over the degree and extent of tissue injury. The characterization of the photothermal biological response following laser irradiation depends, however, on the structural level that is targeted.

At the microscopic level, the photothermal process originates from the bulk absorption occurring in molecular vibration–rotation bands or in the vibrational manifold of the lowest electronic excited state, instantaneously followed by subsequent rapid thermalization through nonradiative decay. Since tissue structures may be considered as a complex condensed phase media, rotation is hindered and vibrational amplitudes are more or less damped. Hence, energy levels are not sharp but broadened. The reaction with a target molecule proceeds in two nearly simultaneous steps.

First, the absorption of a photon of energy h*n*, promoting A to a vibronic state A^*. Secondly, an inelastic scattering occurs at 1–100 psec time-scale with a collisional partner M belonging to the surrounding medium. On colliding with A^*, M instantaneously increases its kinetic energy to M' by carrying away the internal energy released by A^*. The microscopic origin of the temperature rise results from the amount of energy released to M. This two-step reaction can be represented as

$$\text{Absorption:} \quad A + h\nu \rightarrow A^* \ \text{(vibronic)}$$

$$\text{Deactivation:} \quad A^* + M(E) \rightarrow A + M(E + DE) \ \text{(thermal)}$$

For completeness, it should be mentioned that in standard thermodynamic conditions, the kinetic energy per molecule, kT, is about 0.025 eV whereas so-called thermal lasers such as CO_2, Nd:YAG, and argon, have corresponding photon energies 5 to 100 times larger (CO_2: $\lambda = 10.6\ \mu m$, e = 0.12 eV; Nd:YAG: $\lambda = 1.064\ \mu m$, e = 1.17eV; Ar: $\lambda = 514$ nm, e = 2.4 eV).

The photophysical parameter of interest is the absorption coefficient α (cm^{-1}), which also measures the characteristic absorption length $1/\alpha$. This wavelength or frequency dependent coefficient $\alpha(n)$ is the product of the molecular absorption cross-section σ (cm^2) and the number density n (number of homogeneously distributed absorbing molecules per unit volume measured in cm^3)

$$\alpha(\nu) = \sigma n$$

The quantity σnl is the absorbance. A more commonly used form of this law is I $= I_0 10^{\varepsilon(\nu)cl}$ where $\varepsilon(\nu)$, measured in $LMol^{-1}cm^{-1}$, is the molar (decadic) extinction coefficient characteristic of each molecular species in a given solvent and c (mol/L) is the concentration of the absorbing substance.

The absorption of tissue in the UV varies drastically depending on the concentration of DNA and aromatic residues of proteins but in general most organic molecules absorb very strongly in this range. The water absorption coefficient which typically reaches 106 cm^{-1} in the vacuum UV at 100 nm, exhibits a dramatic cut off around 190 nm and has no significant absorption throughout the entire UV range. For physiologic saline, absorption starts below about 200 nm, reaching $\varepsilon \sim 300$ 1/mol-cm at 193 nm, the wavelength of the ArF excimer laser. This absorption is however, due to chlorine ions. Nucleic acids which constitute about 10% to 15% of a cell's dry weight are the most widespread absorbers in 190-300 nm spectral regions. Infrared radiation, on the other hand is absorbed mainly by water with increasingly stronger bands towards longer wavelengths (300 cm^{-1} at 3 μm), with typical absorption depths as small as 10 μm in the far-IR. Between 600 nm and 1,200 nm, radiation penetrates into tissue with low losses due to weaker scattering and absorption and hence reaches deep targets.

The first mechanism by which tissue is thermally affected is molecular denaturation (e.g., proteins, collagen, lipids and haemoglobin). Table 3.2 summarizes the temperature ranges of successive transformations.

Table 3.2 Histological changes in photothermal processes (Conversion of electromagnetic radiation into heat elevation of tissue temperature)

Temperature	**Effects**
43°C–45°C	Conformational changes, retraction, hyperthermia (cell mortality)
50°C	Reduction of enzyme activity
60°C	Protein denaturation, coagulation
80°C	Collagen denaturation, membrane permeabilisation, carbonisation
100°C	Vaporisation and ablation

In the neighbourhood of T ~ 45 °C (hyperthermic range), one observes a tissue retraction related to macromolecular conformational changes, bond destructions and membrane alterations. The range of protein denaturation is between 50°C and 60°C.

As the molecule reaches its "melting temperature", the densely packed polynucleotide chain unfolds and a process called "chain melting" occurs which is associated with a marked increase in light absorption around 260 nm.

Above the protein denaturation temperature, coagulation, necrosis and vacuolation are produced. The temperature limit at which tissues become carbonized is about 80°C. Vaporization occurs beyond 100°C, predominantly from heated free water. The high vaporization heat of water (2,530 J/g) is advantageous, since the steam generated carries away excess heat, thereby preventing further temperature increase of adjacent tissue. Vaporization together with carbonization yield decomposition of tissue constituents. The major problem with material removal is to adjust the duration of laser exposure in order to minimize tissue injury and thermal damage to adjacent zones so as to obtain little necrosis. The scaling parameter for this time-dependent problem is the so-called thermal relaxation time τ, associated with a characteristic diffusion length L. From heat diffusion theory, this latter quantity can be shown to be proportional to the square root of time together with a lumped physical parameter, the tissue diffusivity K(cm^2/sec), characterizing the material thermal response (thermal conductivity, specific heat and density). The relaxation time is then related to L through a relationship of the form $L^2 = 4\,KT$.

For example, since the thermal diffusivity of water is $K = 1.43 \times 10^{-3}\, cm^2/sec$, heat diffuses approximately to 0.8 mm in 1 sec in aqueous media. Similarly, typical thermal relaxation times associated with 10 μm vessels are of the order of 2×10^{-4} sec, whereas for microvasculature of 100 μm size it is approximately 1.8×10^{-2} sec. The relationship serves as the theoretical basis of a scheme, called selective photothermolysis, making use of pulsed irradiation to confine thermally mediated radiation damage to choose pigmented targets at the ultrastructural, cellular or tissue structural level. In the clinical procedure, coagulation and/or vaporization of the tissue must be obtained with minimum thermal damage to the nonirradiated healthy tissue. This requires a precise control of the temperature rise in the irradiated volume and in the surrounding zones. The temperature in the irradiated volume must reach the coagulation or vaporization limit while it must remain below the irreversible damage limit in the untreated tissue. By adjusting the duration of the exposure to the light beam, its energy content and the repetition rate, the temperature rise in the irradiated volume and in the adjacent zones can be controlled in a sufficiently precise way.

If the pulse duration is much shorter than the characteristic time *t* then the heat to diffuse along a length is nearly equal to the penetration depth $1/\alpha$ of the optical radiation. Hence, the optical energy of the pulse is trapped in a volume s/a (s-beam cross section) where it produces a high temperature increase. The expression of *t* is given by

$$\tau = 1/4k\alpha^2$$

For example, for water $k = 1.4 \times 10^{-3}$ cm^2/s (approximately heat diffuses 0.8 cm in 1 sec), heat of vaporization is 2530 J/g at $\lambda = 10.6\ \mu m$ (CO_2 laser), for $\alpha = 10^3$ cm^{-1}; $1/\alpha = 10\ \mu m$; and thus $t = 179\ \mu s$.

Consequently, by pulsing the laser with pulse shorter than 179 μs, it is possible to vapourise tissue directly.

Typical pulse of 10 mJ/50 μs from a CO_2 laser operating at 50 Hz would vaporise 300 μm spots and would cut with a velocity larger than 10 mm/s.

The following Table 3.3 summarises the laser radiation interaction with tissues under photothermal conditions (above threshold intensity).

Table 3.3 Laser radiation interaction with tissues under photothermal conditions (above threshold intensity)

Photothermal interaction	**Effects**
Laser hyperthermia	Condition of elevated tissue temperature below coagulation threshold (40–50^{0}C)
	Enzyme activation
	Cancer therapy
	Laser thermal keratoplasty
	Uniform heating to 70–80^{0}C avoiding shrinkage

Tissue weldings/Anastomoses	Irreversible damage induced by prolonged temperature rise in tissues (50–100^{0}C)
	Permanent denaturation of proteins Tissue whitening and shrinkage
	Body response—dead tissue removal (not under control)
Coagulation	Coagulation of blood vessels up to effective sealing
	Deliberate coagulation and death of target tissue
Haemostasis	Tissue removal through conversion into gaseous vapour (T > 100^{0}C) cutting
Necrosis	
	Endoscopy optical fibre + suction tube Reduces bleeding due to haemostasis Heat conduction thermal time constant *t*
	Surgical precision and control trades off with haemostasis (λ-dependent)
Vaporisation	
	Fast water heating, explosive phase transition and mechanical disruption
Selective photothermolysis	Selection of wavelength and pulsed duration to limit heating to specific structure (dermatological removal of tattoos or pigmented lesions)

3.2.2 Photochemical Interactions

Light may act as a reactant in a photochemical reaction. In this case, the photon energy excites a particular chromophore in a complex biological process, the final outcome of which has a therapeutic relevance. The two processes under photochemical reactions are:

1. Reactions in which molecules are involved as energy carriers or as catalytic regulators after experiencing a photo excitation. In this case the chromophore receptors are said to be photoactivated. One of the most attractive applications of this type is laser spectral sensitisation in which photodynamic therapy (PDT) of malignant tumours appears to be a highly promising technique.

2. Reactions in which the chromophore molecules are modified and converted into photoproducts. An example of general importance is the photoinactivation caused by short-wavelength ultraviolet light used in the recently introduced technique of photoablative microsurgery.

A chromophore compound capable of causing light-induced reactions in molecules that do not absorb light in the same wavelength range is known as a photosensitizer. Following resonant excitation by a monochromatic source, the photosensitizer undergoes a series of simultaneous or sequential decays which result in intramolecular transfer reactions. The decays may ultimately culminate in the release of highly reactive cytotoxic species that cause, irreversible oxidation of some essential cellular components and destroy affected host tissues. The essence of this photochemical interaction is photosensitized oxidation, due to the exogenous chromophore receptor which basically acts as a photocatalyst. It is first activated by resonant absorption, thereby storing energy in one of its excited states. When it deactivates, a chain reaction takes place with a reactant that is not the photosensitizer. Typical photosensitizers are haematophorphyrin derivatives (HpD). The wavelength choice is red radiation 600–700 nm which penetrates deeply in the tissue.

The photochemical interaction involves low-intensity and wavelength-selective lasers.

Wavelength	**Photochemical interaction**
200–315 nm	1. Cells and tissues absorb strongly. 2. Unspecific excitation of many subsystems.
315–400 nm	1. Limited absorption by biomolecules. 2. Some specific absorptions.

400–1000 nm	1. Little absorption by biomolecules. 2. Human cells and tissues are transparent except for red blood cells. 3. Act as optical window between 600-1000 nm.
> 1000 nm	All biomolecules have specific and strong vibrational absorption bands.

The possible sequence of events following exposure of skin to non-ionising radiation leads to beneficial and/or adverse effects as follows:

Chromophore → photochemistry → photoproducts → altered cell function → mediators → biologic responses → beneficial effects and/or adverse effects

Photochemical interactions	Effects
Photochemical ablation	Direct break of chemical bonds leads to tissue ablation No thermal injury Surface is smooth in photochemical interaction High surgical control Less than 5eV power is sufficient

3.2.3 Photomechanical (Photodisruptive) Interactions

It is the mechanical interaction of the target with the acoustic wave associated to the transient absorption of pulsed radiation. This type of effect becomes significant even at 1-10 J/cm causing a characteristic vacuolisation and rupture of the tissue structure. The physical principles lying behind laser-induced breakdown are 1) short laser pulse focussed at target, 2) high power density, 3) high electric field, 4) dielectric breakdown (multiphoton process), 5) plasma formation (free electron), 6) spherical shock wave propagating at low velocity and 7) localised mechanical rupture for small radius.

Basically laser pulse determines a plasma formation via, a laser-induced breakdown. This sudden plasma formation couples a substantial energy to a spherical shock wave propagating into surrounding media. If the irradiation site is submerged into water, the shock wave cannot expand freely and a strong recoil force is transmitted through the tissue bulk. If this force overcomes the strength linking together different portions of a composite structure such as a urinary calculus, it becomes possible to obtain a fragmentation in smaller pieces. This is known as lithotripsy and is entirely neglecting on the excitation of a photomechanical interaction process. In photomechanical interaction, a high power pulsed laser is used to generate a fast high pressure sound wave which causes a mechanical impulse to the tissue. It special features are the following:

a) High laser power densities,

b) Short pulse duration ($d\tau = 10^{-6}$ to 10^{-9} s),

c) Light concentration to small spot (focussing or fibre guiding), and

d) Disruptive effect limited to surroundings of target point.

The conversion mechanisms are as follows:

When ($d\tau > 1\mu s$) a short absorption in target tissue is required or an absorbing mechanical transducer is provided; when $d\tau < 10$ ns, laser-initiated optical breakdown occurs. This causes plasma formation and inverse bremsstrahlung absorption occurs. This leads to expansion of tissue and causes cavitation, finally tissue disrupts. The photodisruptive interactions can be used in lithotripsy, calcified tissue ablation and tumour disruption.

3.2.4 Photoablative Interaction

As already stated, UV radiations are very strongly absorbed by most biomolecules specifically in a band extending from 200 nm to 320 nm. Table 3.2 presents the sequences of effects induced by UV radiation and leading to photodissociation and the release of molecular scale fragments called ablation. Because of the high quantum energy of UV radiation (6.2 to 4 eV), it can modify and even convert chromophores into photoproducts by photodissociation of functionally important compounds such as proteins, nucleic acids, enzymes and pigments.

This feature has recently been exploited experimentally to produce a well-defined, photoablative cut of very small width (50 μm) by exposure to excimer lasers at several UV wavelengths (ArF - 193 nm , 6.4 eV; KrF - 248 nm, 5 eV; XeCl - 308 nm, 4.3 eV), with short pulses (15 ns) focused on various tissues (cornea, skin, plaques). Similar sharp cuts (2.3 μm) with minimal thermal damage are also obtained with the third harmonic of the Nd: YAG laser at 266 nm (4.7 eV), with excellent cutting aspect owing to the high spatial quality of the beam. Control of thermal damage is clinically important since it generally produces undesirable biological effects.

Ablative photodecomposition is a new technique to make a controlled depth and shape in defined areas of specific tissue or body structure and to remove any amount of tissue by ablating that tissue to a predetermined depth. True ablative photodecomposition needs the employment of lasers emitting high peak power UV radiation. In this spectral region, laser ablation produces a trench with sharp and clearly, defined boundaries by light microscopy. Among the various ophthalmological applications, the application for refractive keratoplasty is of great interest as the cornea can be reshaped to correct the most moderate degrees of hyperopia, myopia, and astigmatic defects.

Table 3.4 Physical principles of laser photoablation

Nature	**Effect**
Short UV laser pulse (10 ns) focused on tissue	1–10 W/cm
Strong absorption in the UV (6 eV)	Absorption (proteins:amides:peptides), depth penetration to repulsive
Photodissociation	Excited state

Table 3.5 gives the different threshold observed to ablate a typical tissue with the available excimer laser lines. It is interesting to notice that UV photoablation is

inherently a pulsed process of 100 ns for minimal thermal conduction from the irradiated zone to the bulk.

In general, photoablation is a process which removes biological material with specific issues such as,

1. great depth control because each pulse etches only a few tens of microns
2. a very limited part of the incoming energy is channelled into heat so that a limited rise of temperature take place at the border and
3. very clean and sharp edges, cuts or holes can be obtained in almost all types of tissues with ultraviolet lasers.

Table 3.5 Threshold to ablate a typical tissue with excimer and other lasers

Laser ablation threshold (J/cm)	**Wavelength (nm)**	**Penetration depth (μm)**	**Limiting repetition (Hz)**
ArF (0.05)	193	1	37,000
KrF (0.4)	248	15	156
XeCl (1.3)	308	50	15
Dye	465, 384	8.3	10
Nd:YAG	1.064, 1.400	83	37
Er:YAG (0.05)	2.940	2	9.260
CO_2 (0.5)	10.600	20	93

3.2.5 Biostimulation

The low power laser irradiation can speed up regenerative process in tissues such as wound healing or it can also be an effective therapy in the management of arthritis. The biochemical and physiological mechanism are not understood in pain relief involving biostimulation. The experimental variables in these phenomena are not clear. Further the controlled studies to understand biostimulation are different and controversial and end results tend to be subjective. Until today no rigorous and firm conclusions are drawn about the claims of biostimulation.

3.3 BIOLOGICAL MOLECULES AND TISSUES

1. **Water** It offers an excellent transmission in the region 400 to 800 nm. It gives high absorption peak in the mid-infrared region (1450, 1930, 2940 nm). Water is present in all soft and hard tissues, for example, in skin—70%, cartilage—75%, arteries—80%, bone—10–30%.

2. **Haemoglobin** It has wide diffusion in all tissues except cartilage and dental tissues. It strongly absorbs blue and green haemoglobin absorbs red radiation.

3. **Blood** It is composed of water and haemoglobin. Blood absorbs the optical radiation three times higher at 1064 nm wavelength than 1320 nm wavelength.

4. **Melanin** The biological pigment of skin and other soft tissues contain melanin which absorbs from 1000 to 400 nm.

5. **Xanthophyll** Xanthophyll are the pigments localised in neural fibre layers (for example, macula). It strongly absorbs blue radiation at 460 nm.

6. **Carbon** While heating tissue in the presence of oxygen charring develops carbon. This is due to inflammatory response which is undesired. Carbon strongly absorbs radiation at all wavelengths. It can alter surgical precision. The carbon formation can be minimized with suitable CW lasers.

7. **Collagen** Collagen is the structural component of most tissue. Under mild heating they become sticky (welding and anastomoses) and expend to coagulation (haemostasis). It absorbs infrared radiation at 3030 nm strongly.

8. **Blood vessels** They are hollow soft tissues which are effectively cooled by blood flow. Haemostasis coagulation of proteins in blood increases viscosity and denatures collagen. Haemostasis improves with high power density and longer pulse duration of laser and deeper penetrating wavelengths.

9. Cartilage It consists of water and collagen

10. Bone Bone is a composite material consisting of collagen matrix, calcium phosphate and hydroxyapatite.

11. Dental tissue It consists of enamel dentin, cementum, dental plaque, caries, water, collagen and hydroxyapatite.

12. Atherosclerotic plaque It is a soft plaque deposit composed of fibrous plaque fatty deposit, collagen calcified plaque fatty deposit, and calcium phosphate. It shows low absorption in the visible-near infrared region (white-yellowish colour).

13. Calculus It is strong like deposit of inorganic salts and organic materials accumulated in organs, glands, and ducts. There are great varieties in pigmentation and hence they have wide mechanical properties. Calcium oxalate is very hard while uric acid is hard but not brittle.

3.4 RADIATION DELIVERY SYSTEMS

For every laser source proposed for a biomedical application, it is of outstanding importance to rely on a suitable beam delivery system. The system should be convenient to utilise the laser energy at the site of the irradiation by preserving all the necessary characteristics of the beam. In other words, main requirements for a delivery system are:

1) Good transmission efficiency,

2) Good beam focusability, and

3) Ease in manipulation.

In this respect, both free or guided propagation can provide adequate solutions.

3.4.1 Optical Fibres

In practice, optical fibres constitute an almost ideal solution in terms of transmission efficiency, compactness, flexibility, low cost and so on. The only limitation is due to the typical transmission window for each material constituting the core of the fiber. In silica fibres, reasonable transmission is obtained in the range 0.25-2 mm. A good research has been done to develop IR fibres for transmission in the range 2-10 mm. ZrF and other fluoride glasses are proposed near 3 mm. Thallium and silver halides have been proposed for 10 mm, even if the former is highly toxic. The fibres should deliver maximum power and energy delivery when coupled with laser without causing a permanent and catastrophic damage. CW lasers in this respect do not suffer this damage limitations because very high CW power can be easily transmitted through suitable fibres. This is the case for Nd:YAG lasers which can easily transmit 100 W and more through a 600 mm fibres. Similar situation can be seen in Ar ion lasers, especially for medical applications where much lower power is needed.

Problems have been observed for pulsed lasers. In fact, the very high peak power exerted by Q-switch operation can rise the instantaneous power density at the entrance face of the fibres up to 4 W/cm. This leads to a surface breakdown due to a severe acoustic and thermal damage and ultimately breaks the fibre. Sometimes, high quality beams impinging a fibre with a power density lower than the damage can cause problems inside the bulk of the fibre because of internal reflections. Another class of effects which can cause permanent damage to the fibres is due to the powerful shock wave excited on the target in a liquid environment (opaque or transmitting).

3.4.2 Articulated Arms

For laser emitting out of the range 0.25-2 mm it is possible to use an articulated arm to provide both high transmission efficiency and a reasonable ease to manipulate the beam. A typical articulated arm has 6 arms and rotating joints. This type of articulated arm is typical of surgical CO_2 laser. Figure 3.4 presents two typical articulated arms.

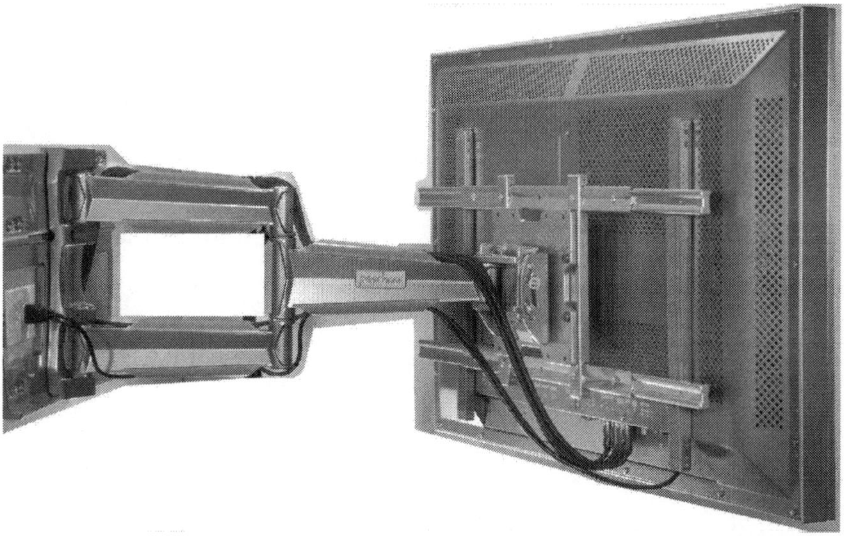

(a)

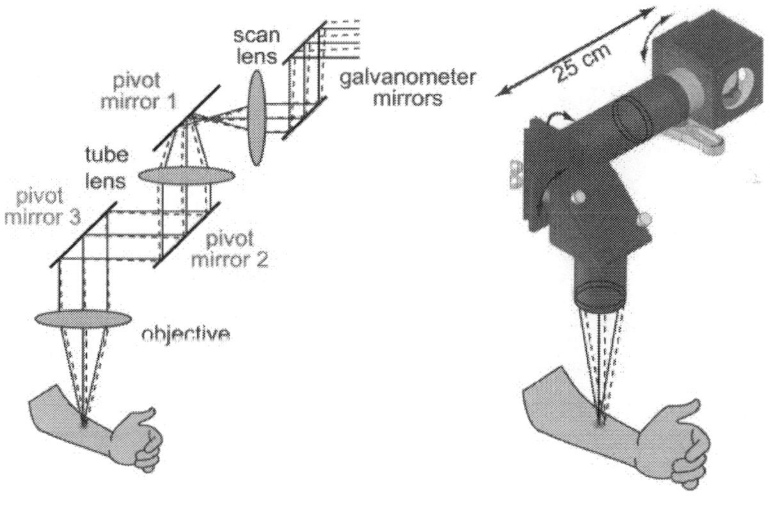

(b)

Figure 3.4 (a) and (b) Two typical articulated arm (Couresy-OSApublishing.org)

References

1. Q. Peng et al. 2008. "Lasers in medicine". Reports on Progress in Physics. 71:056701.

2. J. L. Boulnois. (1986)A. "Photophysical Processes in Recent Medical Laser Developments: a Review". Lasers in Medical Science. 1:47-66

3. A.L. McKenzie. 1990. "Review article: Physics of thermal processes in laser-tissue interaction". Physics in Medicine and Biology. 35(9):1175-1209

4. M.H. Niemz. 2004. Laser-Tissue Interactions. Third, Revised Edition, Springer-Verlag

5. G. Paltauf and P.E. Dyer. 2003. "Photomechanical Processes and Effects in Ablation". Chemical Reviews. 103:487-518

6. P.N. Prasad. 2003. Introduction to Biophotonics. Wiley Inter-Science

7. Cammarata. F. and Wautelety. M. 1999. Medical lasers and laser-tissue interactions. Phys Educ. 34:156–61.

8. A. Vogel and V. Venugopalan. 2003. "Mechanisms of Pulsed Ablation of Biological Tissues". Chemical Reviews. 103:577-644

9. A.J. Welch and M.J.C. van Gemert. Eds. 1995. Optical-Thermal Response of Laser-Irradiated Tissue. Plenum Press. 64

4

Lasers in Dentistry

Dr. Bikash Jyoti Borthakur

Dept. of Conservative Dentistry & Endodontics,

Mahatma Gandhi Postgraduate Institute of Dental Sciences,

Indira Nagar, Puducherry

Dr. S. Mohan

Vel Tech University,

Chennai – 600 062

INTRODUCTION

"Laser" was introduced by Theodor. H. Maimanin in the form of ruby laser at Hughes Research Laboratories in Malibu, California on 16th May 1960. Application of laser in the field of dentistry started when he had exposed an extracted tooth to the invented laser in the same year. Although there have been improvements and developments in this field of science which resulted into its application in wide range of fields including medicine, it took almost 30 years for major breakthrough to happen. With the advent of CO_2, Nd:YAG, Er:YAG, and Er:Cr:YSGG lasers in mid-90s, for hard and soft tissue procedures there have been many studies on applications of lasers since then.

LASER is not supposed to be a "magic wand", still each and every field of medicine utilizes the benefits of laser and dentistry is not an exception.

True research on application of laser in dentistry began when Ralph H Stern and Reider F Sognnaes (1963) of Los Angeles School of Dentistry, University of California studied thermal effects of ruby laser on dental hard tissues and restorative materials. Since then there had been attempts to utilize the benefits of laser in each and every field of dentistry. Laser may be used in dentistry effectively for their ability to incise, cut and ablate soft and hard tissues.

In 1965, Leon Goldman reported the first case of laser exposure to a vital human tooth. One of the reasons of odontophobia or dentophobia of the patients is due to the screeching and annoying noise of the dental tooth cutting tool. There have been attempts to replace dental drills as early as 1945 when Dr Robert Black used air abrasion technology for tooth preparation. It did not get momentum that time as the materials demand precise cavity preparation. Heat, vibration and pressure are the primary causes of fear and pain associated with the use of the traditional dental drill. These are again some of the reasons of patient's unacceptance. Quest to replace a dental drill started with air abrasion technique and ended with application of hard tissue laser. With the advent of dental hard tissue laser, odontophobia was considerably reduced. Since cutting both hard and soft tissues with the laser does not generate heat, vibration or pressure they are widely used in most of the disciplines of dentistry.

Many dental procedures can be performed in a single visit without anesthesia and pain with just fewer pulses of laser.

CLASSIFICATION OF LASER

Laser can be classified as follows:

I. Based on Wavelengths of Light

1. Infrared
2. Visible
3. Ultraviolet

The wavelength is the physical distance covered by one cycle of a sinusoidal wave. Wavelengths of dental laser lie in different light zones, from long wavelength (infrared, e.g., $CO_{2,}$Nd:YAG, Er:YAG, Er,Cr:YSGG, etc.) and visible wavelength (e.g., He:Ne, Argon) to short wavelength (ultraviolet, e.g., excimer) regions which are non-ionising and non-mutagenic radiations.

II. Dental Lasers May also be Grouped According to Output Level

1. Low output or soft tissue lasers

2. High output or hard tissue lasers

The output level is the energy per second measured in watts emitted from the laser in the form of coherent light. The rate of energy delivery is expressed in watts (Joules per second). In diode lasers, there is a semiconductor device that produces coherent radiation that require only a few milli watts of power at 3 to 12 volts DC and several milli amperes thus, small battery can be used for power supply. It is also known as an injection laser in the visible or infrared (IR) spectrum when current passes through it. As it is of low output, dental diode lasers are also known as soft tissue lasers.

III. According to the Active Medium

1. Solid-state

2. Gas

3. Dye

An active medium is the material used (solid, gas or dye) to emit the laser light and after which the laser is named. Excimer is an abbreviation for *excited dimer*. A mixture of gas is used as the active medium in a family of lasers emitting ultraviolet light.

IV. According to the Oscillation Mode

1. Continuous wave

2. Pulsed wave

Laser which delivers energy in the form of a single or train of pulses. A laser emitting for a period in excess of 0.25 second is known as continuous wave laser. Pulsed wave is not continuous and can be used by producing independent free running pulses or by interrupting a continuous wave by gated or chopped pulse.

IV. According to American National Standard Institute and Occupational Health and Safety Administration (OSHA)

Lasers are classified as:

- Class I: Low-powered laser that are safe to use, e.g., laser pointer, UPC scanner
- Cass II a: Low-powered visible lasers that are hazardous if viewed directly for more than 1000 seconds, e.g., laser printer, CD, DVD and BD player and reader
- Class II b: Low-powered visible lasers that are hazardous if viewed directly for more than 0.25 seconds.
- Class III a: Medium-powered lasers that are normally hazardous if viewed directly for less than 0.25 seconds without magnifying optics.
- Class III b: Medium-powered lasers that can be hazardous if viewed directly. Use of a Class 3 laser requires special training and eye protection. One example of a Class 3 laser would be a dental argon curing light.
- Class IV: High-powered lasers (> 0.5 W) that can produce ocular, skin and fire hazards.

Most of the dental lasers belong to Class IV category. Therefore, proper laser protective measures are mandatory for dentists as well as patients.

Laser–tissue interaction is nothing but photonic absorption within tissue's chromophores. Parts of the tissue that absorb laser light energy are termed as chromophores. Oral tissues contain several chromophores, e.g., melanin, hemoglobin, other pigmented proteins, hydroxyapatite and water. Generally, visible or NIR (near infrared) wavelengths of lasers will be absorbed better by pigmented tissues whereas non-pigmented tissues absorb longer wavelengths of lasers. This increases tissue temperature very rapidly to evaporative state. When these lasers cut tissue, it is known as photothermal interaction or photothermal ablation. In laser–tissue interaction, the two independent parameters are:

- Laser wavelength, and
- Inherent quality of tissue.

The control that is in dentist's hand is:

- Control power density,
- Total power delivered over a given surface area,
- The rate and duration of exposure, and
- The mode of delivery.

During ablation, colour change of the tissue can be observed and at that point laser tip should be moved in "paint brush motion" to get optimal result. Instead, if fast and constant painting motion is applied on the tissue, proper ablation will not occur.

In most lasers, excisional or incisional operations are accompanied at 100^{0}C where vaporization of intracellular and extracellular water causes ablation. If the temperature exceeds by 200^{0}C during laser procedure, carbonization and irreversible tissue necrosis will occur. That is why low power is selected to complete successful operation.

For selecting lasers for dentistry, coagulation, sterilization and biostimulatory effects of lasers are considered the most. The following lasers with their corresponding wavelength are commonly used for soft and hard tissue applications in dentistry. The lasers function with an *end cutting* action while other dental instruments are *side cutting*.

Table 4.1 Properties of Lasers Used in Dentistry

Laser	Type	Power	Wave length(nm)	Mode	Tissue interaction	Delivery System
Diode	Infrared (IR), Solid (S)	Up to 100 W	812	Pulsed (P), Continuous wave (CW),	Photoablation	Fiber optic
Nd:YAG	IR, Solid (S)	Average 6 W	1064,1300	CW	Photothermal Photo-disruption	Fiber optic
Nd:YAG	IR, S	Average 6 W	1064	P	Photothermal Photo-disruption	Fiber optic
CO_2	IR, Gas (G)	25 W-320 W	10600	CW	Photothermal	Mirror system
CO_2	IR,G	4-10 W	10600	P	Photothermal	Mirror system
Er:YAG	IR, S	6,5 W	2940	P	Photothermal Photoablation	Mirror system
Er,Cr:YSGG	IR, S	175 mW-350 mW	2780, 2940	CW, P	Photoablation	Fiber optic
KTP	Visible (V),S	1.5 W-3 W	532	CW	Photoablation	Fiber optic
Ho:YAG	IR, S	2.0 W	2060, 2120	P	Photothermal Photoablation	Fiber optic
He Ne	V, G	0.1-10 mW	633,1152	CW	Biostimulation	Fiber optic

Laser	Type	Power	Wave length(nm)	Mode	Tissue interaction	Delivery System
Excimer	UV, D	25-100 mW	190-351	P	Photoablation	Fiber optic, mirror system
Argon	V, G	20 W	488,514	CW	Photothermal	Fiber optic
Ti:Sapphire	V, G	0.1-1W	700-1100	CW, tunable	Photothermal	Fiber optic
GaAIAs	IR	20 mW	780	CW	Photobiostimulation	Cylindrical quartz tip

Table 4.2 Use of Lasers in Different Branches of Dentistry

Branch		CO_2	Excimer	Nd:YAG	Argon	HeNe	Ho:YAG	Er:YAG	GaAIAs	KTP	Diode	Ti:Sapphire	Er,Cr:YSGG
Oral Surgery	Coagulation & cutting excision	√		√	√	√	√				√		
	Surgical removal of Hemangiomas, papilloma, fibroma, mucocele, etc.	√		√			√				√		
	Lingual frenectomy						√						

Branch		CO_2	Excimer	Nd:YAG	Argon	HeNe	Ho:YAG	Er:YAG	GaAIAs	KTP	Diode	Ti:Sapphire	Er,Cr:YSGG
Periodontics	Gingivectomy	√	√	√		√	√	√			√		√
	Excision												
	Calculus removal							√				√	
	Scaling & root planning			√							√		
	Peri-implantitis							√			√		
	Hyperpigmentation										√		
	LANAP			√									
	Osseous surgery							√					√
Conservative Dentistry & Endodontics	Root canal disinfection	√	√	√				√			√		√
	Bleaching									√	√		
	Caries diagnosis, prevention & treatment							√					√
	Cavity preparation							√					√
	Etching							√					
	Photopolymerization				√								
	Rest and removal							√					
	Desensitization							√					

Branch		CO_2	Excimer	Nd:YAG	Argon	HeNe	Ho:YAG	Er:YAG	GaAlAs	KTP	Diode	Ti:Sapphire	Er,Cr:YSGG
Prosthodontics	Pre-prosthetic surgeries	√			√						√		
	Tooth preparation							√					√
	Gingival retraction	√			√			√			√		
	Modification pontic design, etc.							√					
	Laminate removal							√					
Pedodontics	Same laser can be used as applicable to the surgical, conservative & endodontic, orthodontic procedures related to children.												
Orthodontics	Tooth movement								√				
	Laser welding			√	√				√				
Oral Medicine	i) Excisional biopsy—leucoplakia, sq.cell carcinomas		√			√							
	ii)Holography				√	√							
	iii)Optical Coherent Tomography												
	iv) Irradiation of aphthous stomatitis, non-erosive lichen planus, Herpes								√		√		
	v)TMJ dysfunction syndrome								√		√		
	vi)Myofacial pain dysfunction syndrome								√		√		

N.B.-These are some of the specialty-wise uses of laser. This is not the complete list.

Each wavelength, power output, energy density, delivery device and mode have its own unique interactive qualities and laser operator's skill plays a major role in making laser as a success tool in dentistry.

ADVANTAGES OF LASER

Oral and maxillofacial surgery was the forerunner in using laser. There were attempts to replace surgical scalpel with electrocautery and later with laser. Some of the added advantages of laser are:

- Better haemostasis,
- Controlled depth of penetration,
- Reduced pain,
- Reduced post-operative edema,
- Dry operating field,
- Excellent visibility,
- Suture may not be needed,
- Decreased scarring,
- Enhanced healing,
- Improved coagulation,
- Rapid regeneration,
- Less chances of metastasis, and
- Sterilization of treatment site and no infection.

APPLICATIONS OF LASER

1. Oral and Maxillofacial Surgery

Following are some of the applications of laser in oral and maxillofacial surgery.

1. Excision as well as excisional biopsy of pathological lesions like leukoplakia and squamous cell papilloma.
2. Incision and drainage.
3. Surgical removal of benign lesions in the form of a fibroma or a papilloma on the lip, tongue, buccal mucosa or palatal area.
4. Removal of tongue lesions and hemiglossectomy, etc.
5. Coagulation of bleeding areas and soft tissue graft donor site.
6. Ablation of an intraosseous dental pathology such as granulation tissue or an abscess.
7. Surgical removal of squamous cell carcinomas.
8. Treating heamorrhagic diathesis.
9. Haemangiomas.
10. Apical root resection.
11. Coagulation of extraction sites.
12. Surgical extraction of impacted teeth and other teeth with less traumatic flaps and bone removal.
13. Ankyloglossia.

Ankyloglossia is seen in many adolescent patients (attachment of heavy lingual frenum). Micropulsed CO_2 lasers (for ablation of soft tissues) with char-free settings (30 Hz, 300 mJ) was used to achieve minimal collateral thermal damage in ankylogossia. There was a little or no bleeding during surgery and suturing was contraindicated as healing takes place in advance[120]. It was reported that the speech improved dramatically after surgery.

CO_2 lasers have been popular in oral surgery due to their precise incisions and excellent hemostasis. It is a commonly used laser for incisional & excisional biopsies[121, 122].

One of the advantages of CO_2 in removing malignant lesion from oral cavity is being minimal bleeding, less postoperative pain, precise cancer diode surgery and minimal metastasis. Indicated power setting ranges from 4–10 W.

Due to its biostimulative properties, Nd:YAG can be used to promote healing, improve osteogenesis, and give post-operative comfort to the patient. In case of bleeding from an extraction socket, Nd:YAG lasers can be used to form fibrin rapidly thereby creating a quick and more durable clot.

Besides photopolymerization of composite resin, argon laser can be used for excision of traumatic hemangioma also.

Er:YAG laser can be used for removal of large benign oral lesion without placement of sutures (Keller et al 1990). Erbium lasers are capable of cutting bone in a less traumatic fashion and can be quite useful in oral surgical procedures. It is the unique laser that can cut both hard and soft tissues.

Dental lasers can be used in the treatment of bisphosphonate-induced osteonecrosis of the jaw (BONJ). BONJ occurs because the drug inhibits osteoclastic activity. When Er:YAG laser is used to remove the necrotic bone, the remaining bone is traumatized minimally so that osteoclastic activity is minimized. Nd:YAG biostimulation can also be used concurrently or separately to promote bone healing as well. Recent studies have shown superior results when compared to traditional surgical approaches when lasers are used.

2. Periodontics

The scope of use of laser in periodontics is of many-folds.

Laser can be used in periodontics for:

I. Initial Periodontal Therapy Like:

1. Debridement of tooth structure (nonsurgically)
2. Selective removal of calculus
3. Periodontal drug delivery
4. Bacterial reduction from gingival sulcus by host modulation

Soft tissue lasers like argon, Nd:YAG and diode laser are selected for coagulation and bacterial reduction.

II. Periodontal Soft Tissue Surgical Applications Like:

1. Gingivectomy and gingivoplasty
2. Frenectomy
3. Removal of benign tumours like epulis and others
4. Gingival depigmentation
5. Exposure of dental implants in second stage surgery
6. Management of aphthous ulcers
7. Free gingival graft coagulation
8. Crown lengthening

For soft tissue periodontal surgical procedures, the widely used lasers are CO_2, Nd:YAG,diode, Er:YAG and Er,Cr:YSGG. Gingivectomy is the most common procedure performed with dental lasers. All laser wavelengths can be used to precisely incise gingiva for restorative, cosmetic, orthodontic, prosthodontic and periodontal indications. Rapid healing and reduced pain are commonly seen post-operatively and patients rarely need periodontal packing or sutures. The thermal effects of diodes, Nd:YAG and CO_2 lasers must be understood to avoid collateral damage. Erbium lasers by pulsed technology, shallow penetration, and water absorption produces a minimal thermal effect and minor procedures can sometimes be achieved with no anesthetic at all. The nearly "cold cutting" effect of erbium tissue interaction creates a remarkable post-operative course.

III. Root Surface Modifications

For root surface modification and for reattachment, CO_2, Nd:YAG, Er:YAG and diode laser had been attempted.

Recently Laser Assisted New Attachment Procedure (LANAP) showed promising results. By definition LANAP is "*Cementum-mediated new attachment to the root surface in the absence of a long junctional epithelium.*"

In LANAP procedure, without elevating a flap surgically, a thin laser fiber is inserted deep into the periodontal pocket. Selective photothermolysis effect of laser is utilized for removing diseased, infected, and inflamed pocket epithelium while preserving healthy adjacent tissue. Due to precise tissue ablation and laser light, energy is attracted to pigmented tissues and coloured bacteria causing the destruction of periodontal pathogens resulted in antiseptic hemostasis. Hemostasis is finally achieved with a fibrin clot.

There is no need for placement of sutures or surgical glue, closure is relied on the fibrin clot and tissue compression.

IV. Osseous Periodontal Surgery

Er:YAG laser can be a useful tool in osseous periodontal surgery, however, lower cutting efficiency and lack of depth control are few of its limitations.

Nd:YAG and erbium lasers have been the most studied and utilized wavelengths in periodontal therapy. Nd:YAG lasers are useful in periodontics because of their affinity for pigment which allows selective debridement of diseased sulcular epithelium. The Nd:YAG wavelength is also bactericidal, biostimulative, and has the ability to stimulate fibrin formation with the proper parameters. Erbium lasers have been shown to be effective at scaling and root planning, effective pocket decontamination, and can replace scalpels when incisions are needed. One notable advantage to laser techniques is a predictably more comfortable post-operative experience for patients.

Treatment of herpetic and recurrent aphthous ulcer lesions, uncovering of an implant, gingival retraction, ablation of periapical granuloma or an abscess and removal of lesions like fibroma, papilloma on the lip, tongue, buccal mucosa or palate can easily be done with diode lasers.

The diode lasers are efficient soft tissue lasers. The clinical advantages of diode lasers are better hemostasis, ability to seal nerve endings and lymphatic vessels, less post-operative pain and swelling, aids overall healing and sutureless surgery.

It should be remembered that lasers offer unchallenging advantages in precision, cutting and hemostasis. Lomke (2009) used Er:YAG laser to retract the marginal gingival tissues adjacent to finish lines prior to making final impressions for crown and bridge. He used very low energy (1000 micro sapphire tip, 100-200 mJ) with a repetition rate of 12 Hz.

Lasers are also widely used for excision biopsies of benign soft tissue lesions in the oral cavity.

As we know the main chromophore for erbium laser is water. Erbium laser is the only laser that can cut both hard and soft tissues and ablate tooth and bone due to its special absorption qualities. Er:YAG laser has thermomechanical effect which is due to rapid buildup of heat and spontaneous evaporation of the available water content. In certain clinical cases, Er:YAG can be used to remove a defective composite restoration, eradicate recurrent decay and to perform crown lengthening. The Er:YAG laser can also be used effectively for clinical cases that involve full thickness flaps and osseous recontouring.

3. Prosthetic Dentistry and Implantology

Lasers have been used in a variety of procedures in prosthetic dentistry and implantology.

i. Crown lengthening of varied indications.

ii. Soft tissue management of abutments, passively erupted tooth, osteointegrated implants and laminates.

iii. Gingival retraction.

iv. For modification of pontic design.

v. Removal of laminates.

vi. Implant recovery and impression making can be done in a single appointment only if laser is used.

vii. Implant site preparation can be done easily even in patient with blood dyscrarias.

viii. Treatment of deficient alveolar ridges.

ix. Undercut in the alveolar ridges.

x. Treatment of enlarged tuberosity.

xi. Surgical treatment of tori and exostoses, alveoplasty, pre-prosthetic ridge preparation/hyperplasic tissue reduction, tuberosity reductions, vestibuloplasty and tori removal are some of the pre-prosthetic surgeries.

xii. Application of laser in dental laboratory: Laser holographic imaging is a well-established method for storing topographic information, such as tooth preparations, facial forms, occlusal tables, etc. The use of two laser beams allows more complex surface detail to be mapped using interferometry. Laser scanning of casts can be linked to computerized milling equipment for fabrication of restorations from porcelain and other similar materials. Several lasers are used for holographic imaging, e.g., Helium-Neon (He-Ne), Helium-cadmium (He-Cd), Argon-ion (Ar^+) and Krypton-ion (Kr^+) lasers

4. Orthodontic Indications

Lasers can be used in the following orthodontic indications:

i. Aesthetic gingival recontouring.

ii. Exposure of unerupted and partially erupted teeth.

iii. Frenectomies.

iv. Removal of inflamed and hypertrophic tissue.

v. Miscellaneous tissue removal.

vi. Low-intensity laser therapy (LILT) accelerate human teeth movement and could therefore considerably shorten the whole treatment duration.

Frenectomies are very common laser procedures that can be accomplished effectively with any wavelength. Simple ones can often be achieved with topical anesthesia only. Hemostasis is usually excellent, particularly with the more thermal CO_2, Nd:YAG, and diodes.

DIAGNOSTIC LASERS

Imaging soft and hard tissue can be done with Optical Coherence Tomography (OCT). It is an emerging non-invasive imaging modality that takes tomographic images of the hard and soft tissue which have a promising prospect for dentistry. It is very useful to detect demineralization and remineralization in dental caries. OCT is also useful for detection of secondary caries also. It can give resolution of up to 10 μm which is superior to radiography in resolution (up to 10 times). OCT provides detailed characterization of the dental hard and soft structures, enabling dentists to make accurate and early diagnosis of oral diseases including dental caries and periodontal disease.

Titanium:Sapphire laser is a femtosecond ultrafast and accurate laser that can perform hard tissue ablation without any thermal damage of natural tooth structure. It gives precise, clean and superior cutting. It will be an alternative to the mechanical drill and Er:YAG laser. The drawbacks of Er:YAG laser are that it leaves microcracks and causes collateral thermal and/or pulpal damage within tooth. Although Ti:Sapphire is more advantageous, it causes acoustic damage in underlying tissues resulting in microfractures and cracks within the healthy parts of the tooth.

PHOTODYNAMIC THERAPY (PDT)

Photodynamic therapy (PDT) is an effective therapy in treating cancer in general and oral cancer in particular. The advantage of PDT for early carcinomas of the oral cavity is the ability to preserve normal tissues while effectively removing cancerous tissues up to 1 cm in depth. PDT is an effective method for the treatment of dysplastic, invasive types of malignant lesion. Mang et al[128] reported successful treatment of squamous cell carcinoma of palate.

In addition to their surgical capabilities, lasers can be used as very low energy for different clinical conditions. The terms Low Level Laser Therapy (LLLT) or bio-stimulation or "Photo biostimulation" are often used interchangeably to describe this phenomenon. Here low energy density of visible red or near infra-red spectrum of light is used. In dentistry, LLLT can be useful for the following conditions:

- Recurrent aphthous stomatitis and traumatic ulcers
- To alleviate pain after extraction
- Reduction of oral edema
- Post-operative analgesia following oral surgical procedures
- Post-herpetic recurrent herpetic lesion
- TMJ dysfunction syndrome
- Trigeminal neuralgia
- Management of inflammatory conditions such as erosive lichen planus
- Reduce pain of orthodontics
- Enhance healing
- Reducing oedema
- Chronic orofacial pain

LASERS IN PEDODONTICS

Dental lasers offer many advantages when treating pediatric patients. All procedures previously discussed apply to pediatric treatments as well. The ability to provide care with less use of needles and high-speed hand pieces makes it more acceptable and less traumatic to children. Behavioral management improves when these devices are not used as these are one of the causes of anxiety and fear. Subsequent treatment appointments are often easier to manage when the child had more positive experience.

The ability to perform less invasive procedures with greater patient comfort makes laser dentistry more popular to dentists as well as patients. A thorough understanding of laser physics and biological effects is mandatory. Comprehensive and ongoing training is imperative to use these devices effectively and safely.

References

1. Maiman, T.H. 1960. Stimulated optical radiation in ruby. *Nature*. 187:493-494.

2. Leo, J. Miserendino. 1995. History and development of Laser Dentistry: In *Lasers in Dentistry*. Leo, J. Miserendino, Robert, M. Pick. Quintessence Publishing Co.Inc. Singapore.

3. Goldman L. 1991. Background to laser medicine-History, principles and safety. In Goldman (ed): Laser Non surgical Medicine. Lancaster, PA Technomic Publishing Co. Inc.

4. Black, R.B. 1950. Airbrasive: some fundamentals. *J Am Dent Assoc*. 41:701–10.

5. http://www.rli.com/resources/articles/classification.aspx

6. C.Y.Park, S.G.Kim, M.D.Kim, T.G.Eom, A.H.Yoon, S.G.Ahn. 2005. Surface properties of endosseous dental implants after Nd:YAG and CO treatment at various energies. *J.Oral Maxillo fac. Surg*. 63:1522-1527

7. Pecaro, B.C. and Garchume, W.J. 1983. The CO_2 laser in Oral and maxillofacial surgery. *J.Oral Maxillo fac Surg*. 41:725-728

8. Robert, M., Pick, M., Anthony, P. and Loh, H.S. 1995. Clinical application of the CO_2 Laser in "*Laser in dentistry*". Ch.9 p145. Leo, J. Miserendino and Robert, M. Pick, Quintessence Publishing Co.Inc.,Singapore.

9. Robert, M., Pick, M., Anthony, P. and Loh, H.S. 1995. Clinical application of the CO_2 Laser in "*Laser in dentistry*". Ch.9 p141. Leo, J. Miserendino and Robert, M. Pick, Quintessence Publishing Co.Inc.,Singapore.

10. Bains V.K., Gupta S. and Bains R. 2010. Lasers in Periodontics: An Overview. *J of oral health and community dentistry.* 4(Spl)

11. Brown S.I. 2013. Current Advances in the Use of Lasers in Periodontal Therapy: A LANAP Case Series. *Clinical Advances in Periodontics*. 1-27.

12. Brown S.I. 2013. Curent advances in the use of Lasers in periodontal therapy: a laser assisted new attachment procedure case series. *Clinical advances in Periodontics*. 3(2) May2013 96-103

13. Lomke, M.A. 2009. Clinical applications of dental lasers. *General dentistry*. 47-59

14. T.S.Mang, M. Sullivan, M.Cooper, T.Loree, N. Rigual. 2006. The use of photodynamic therapy using 630 nm laser light and porlimer sodium for the treatment of oral squamous cell carcinoma. *Photodiag. Photodynam.Ther.* 3:272-275

15. Walsh L. J. 1997. The current status of low level laser therapy in dentistry. Part 1. Soft tissue applications. *Aust Dent J* 42 :(4):247-54.

16. Kaur S., Amin T., Mir S., Nazir S., Abdullah S. Application of Lasers in Prosthodontics IJCCI *2013. 5(1),33:40,2013*

17. Spitz S.D. Lasers in prosthodontics: Clinical realities of a dental laser in a prosthodontic practice. AlphaOmegan 101(4)188-194

18. Cruz D.R., Eduardo K. K., Ribeiro M.S. and Wetter, N.U. 2004. Effects of Low-Intensity Laser Therapy on the Orthodontic Movement Velocity of Human Teeth: A Preliminary Study. *Lasers in Surgery and Medicine*. 35:117–120

5

Laser application in Conservative Dentistry & Endodontics

Dr. Bikash Jyoti Borthakur, M.D.S.

Professor & Head,

Department of Conservative Dentistry & Endodontics,

Mahatma Gandhi Postgraduate Institute of Dental Sciences,

Indira Nagar, Puducherry

5.1 LASER APPLICATION IN CONSERVATIVE DENTISTRY AND ENDODONTICS

Ever since "Laser" was introduced in the form of ruby laser by Theodor Harold Maiman of Hughes Research Laboratories in Malibu, California on 16th May 1960, there have been rapid improvements and developments in this field of science which resulted into its application in wide range of fields including medicine.

Dr. Charles J. Campbell of the Institute of Ophthalmology at Columbia-Presbyterian Medical Center and Charles J. Koester of the American Optical Co. at Columbia-Presbyterian Hospital in Manhattan were credited with performing the first laser treatment. They used ruby laser to destroy a retinal tumor.

Research on application of laser in dentistry began when Ralph H Stern and Reider F Sognnaes (1963) of Los Angeles School of Dentistry, University of California studied thermal effect of ruby laser on dental hard tissues and restorative materials.

In 1965, Leon Goldman first reported the case of laser exposure to a vital human tooth.

Within the last five decades, many types of laser had been introduced after ruby laser ranging from the second laser, uranium laser by Peter P. Sorokin and Mirek Stevenson of the IBM Thomas J. Watson Research Center (November, 1960), helium-neon, neodymium glass (Nd:glass) laser by Elias Snitzer (October, 1961), gallium-arsenide laser, GaAsP (gallium arsenide phosphide) laser diode, carbon-dioxide (CO_2) laser, yttrium aluminum garnet (YAG) laser, Nd:YAG (neodymium-doped YAG) laser, xenon lasers, argon-ion laser, dye laser, excimer laser, free-electron laser (FEL), titanium-sapphire laser, quantum dot laser, the quantum cascade (QC) laser, pulsed atom laser, electrically powered hybrid silicon laser, mode-locked silicon evanescent laser, short-pulse lasers to most recent single atom laser (2010).

Due to rapid progress in the field of laser research and technology, their delivery system, better understanding of laser–tissue interactions, and well-defined safety guidelines, more and more laser have been used in the field of medicine as well as in dentistry. This "magic wand" is the talk of dentistry which resulted into initiation of study club, society for the purpose of sharing and gathering information on Laser by Goal VP as early as in 1989 and by the ADA approved body American Laser Dentist (ALD) in 1993.

Although it is not included in BDS curriculum, there is a need to incorporate it for better understanding at grassroots level of dental education. In India, an affiliate body of ALD, USA was formed in October 2011, by likeminded individuals with the aim to promote laser education in India.

As laser-assisted dentistry is in a very promising stage and there is very rapid progress and advancement in this technology, laser is the future of dentistry.

There are varied applications of laser in each and every field of dentistry. Here are some of the important clinical applications in the branch of "Conservative Dentistry" and "Endodontics".

Application of laser in "Conservative Dentistry"and "Endodontics" can be highlighted for the following purposes:

i. Diagnostic

ii. Preventive

iii. Treatment

APPLICATIONS OF LASER IN THE FIELD OF CONSERVATIVE DENTISTRY

The following are the applications of laser in the field of Conservative Dentistry:

5.2 DIAGNOSTIC

Laser plays a very important role in early detection of incipient enamel caries as well as micro-cracks and incomplete fractures.

1. Laser Transillumination

Regular light source had been used to detect dental caries, tooth fracture and crack as the index of light transmission is lower in comparison to healthy tooth. Bjelkagen et al. (1982) used the luminescence excited by visible argon laser light for early detection of caries. Here, carious structures appear darker than the non-carious one.

Kutsch VK (1992) presented his clinical trial of caries illumination with argon laser in third International Congress on Laser in dentistry. The carious tooth structure was readily apparent with the laser with a clinical appearance of a dark fiery, orange-red colour whereas decalcified areas appear as a dull, opaque orange colour.

The involved tooth can either be illuminated with a beam of blue green light of argon ion laser at wave length of 488 nm from facial or lingual/palatal aspect by keeping the delivery fiber in desired surface and observe from the opposite side. Then laser fluorescence is observed in 540 nm.

Sometimes fluorescence dye (e.g., sodium fluorescein) is incorporated in the involved tooth tissues prior to laser exposure, which will give stronger fluorescence. Laser will often detect dental caries, which is undetectable in radiograph.

5.3 Quantitative Laser Fluorescence (QLF)

Here, same argon ion laser with blue green light of 488 nm wavelength is used. A modified portable version of QLF was made available by Inspector Research System, Netherland with the following components

i) Measuring probe

ii) Control unit

iii) Frame grabber

5.4 Laser Induced Fluorescence

Diagnodent system: These are commercially available laser fluorescence devices (a variant of QLF system). There are two varieties.

i) Diagnodent

ii) Diagnodent pen

Hibst & Gall's (1998) research led to development of Diagnodent in the year 1998. Here, red laser light of 655 nm is used instead of blue light. It recognizes caries by increased fluorescence over sound tooth structure. Source of light is a laser diode in the form of aluminum, gallium, indium and phosphorus (AlGaInP). When laser excites organic components of dental hard tissues, it quantifies the emitted fluorescence. A photo diode measures the amount of fluorescence light passing through the filter. The signal is displayed as an integer of 0-99 with an audible beep.

Diagnodent pen is a handheld compact and portable device without the conventional unit of diagnodent. It requires a clean dry tooth surface. Laser passes through enamel without being deflected as it is more transparent. In case of caries affected enamel, light will get diffracted and dispersed. During the carious process, one of the bacterial metabolic products is porphyrin which is a fluorophore. The laser is able to excite either the dental hard tissue or fluorophores resulting in fluorescence by porphyrins which is collected by nine concentric fibers and translated into numeric values varying from 0-99. There are two optical tips—one for occlusal surface (Tip A) and the other is smooth surface (Tip B). The manufacturer has recommended threshold scores that represent the present and extent of lesion.

Initial lesion Values between 5–25

Early dentinal caries Values just greater than this range

Advanced dentinal caries Values > 35

A restorative intervention is usually considered when diagnodent value is of about 30.

PREVENTION

Laser can be utilized in three ways for prevention of dental caries.

1. By changing the morphological characteristics of enamel
2. By placing pit and fissure sealant by laser curing
3. By inhibiting the cariogenic bacteria

Argon laser can be used to make the surface enamel more caries-resistant by making it less susceptible to caries as well as facilitates the uptake of fluoride by the tooth. Loben RR and Fine S of Forsynth Dental Center, Boston shifted the attention from ruby laser towards CO_2 laser in 1966. When enamel was lased with CO_2, hydroxyapatite was converted to insoluble and impermeable orthocalcium phosphate which helped to reduce subsurface demineralization.

There had been attempts to induce resistance to acid penetration and sealing pit and fissure. Although it can fuse and change the crystalline structure of hydroxyapatite to tricalcium phosphate, there is rise in surface temperature resulting in zones of carbonization and detrimental effect on pulp.

Later low energy CO_2 laser had been used by Stewart et al. (1985) for pit and fissure sealant and by Nelson et al. (1986) for caries prevention but failed to stimulate widespread acceptance due to hazards on pulp.

Excimer laser (Xecl, 308 nm) has bactericidal action against cariogenic bacteria (*S. mutans*). This action is directly related to length of exposure. Nd: YAG laser can also be beneficial in killing *S. mutans*.

TREATMENT

5.3 Photodynamic Therapy (PDT)

In the recent years, photodynamic therapy has emerged as a promising non-invasive treatment modality for infections caused by range of organisms like bacteria, fungi, virus, etc. There are many synonyms used for PTD like photoactive disinfection (PAD), photodynamic antimicrobial therapy (PACT), photodynamic inactivation (PDI), etc.

It can be defined as an oxygen-dependent photochemical reaction that occurs upon light activation of photo sensitizers leading to the generation of cytotoxic reactive oxygen species predominantly singlet oxygen.

Neils Finsen, a Danish physician was credited with the first report on photodynamic therapy. In PDT, to activate the photo sensitizer, a low power light of specific wave length is used. Light source ranges from QTH, LED, plasma arch to lasers like gallium-aluminum-arsenide diode (630-690 nm, 830-906 nm), helium-neon (633 nm) or argon (488-514 nm) laser.

The wavelength ranges from

i. visible to blue in argon laser,

ii. red in helium neon, and

iii. infra-red in diode lasers.

It is a very useful and effective therapeutic technique for prevention and treatment of dental caries.

Araújo et al. (2009) evaluated the antimicrobial effect of PDT against *S. mutans* using red laser in combination with toluidine blue or methylene blue. When they are used at 25 mg/L concentration in association with a red laser, it showed excellent potential to be used in PDT in lethal sensitization of *S. mutans.* PDT can also be used to disinfect carious dentine prior to restoration.

5.4 During Treatment Phase

Different types of lasers are used during different phases of restorative treatment.

5.4.1 *Dental Drill vs Laser* One of the reasons of fear by the dentists (especially for children) even for adults is due to the dental drill. There had been attempts to replace the drill by many means. Hard tissue laser is one of them.

In 1985, Dr. Terry Myers and William Myers developed first true dental laser system (American Dental laser, DL 300, Sunrise Technologies, Inc. Sunnyvale CA) using Nd:YAG laser. They used it for incipient caries removal. It was approved by Food and Drug Administration, USA. Due to the high energy level required to ablate enamel and dentine, CO_2 and Nd:YAD laser causes irreparable pulpal damage and hence now they are not suitable for dental hard tissue removal.

In January 1987, for the first time Food & Drug Administration, USA gave the nod for marketing of CO_2 laser for oral surgical use to Pfizer Laser Co. for a low portable laser unit.

Only a limited number of investigational uses have been approved for the purpose of gathering the necessary information to ensure the safety and efficiency of laser application to dental hard tissue. The following laser system, Er: YAG, Ho: YAG and excimer have the potential to replace the dental drill for cutting enamel, dentine and removal of dental caries. For those lasers whose wavelength is shorter than 2,500 nm can be delivered through an optical fiber system in the form of hand-held piece with air water coolant. Laser hand piece came in a variety of styles and sizes. A laser hand piece should

i) be of light weight,

ii) have a positive gripping surface,

iii) be autoclavable,

iv) be able to accommodate a variety of disposable canulas, and

v) be preferably with fiber locking mechanism and air water spray.

ArF excimer laser (193 nm) can non-thermally ablate calcified dental tissues probably by photo dissociation of organic molecular bonds. Disintegrating effect on dental hard tissue occurs without surface charring and temperature elevation, hence, it can ablate tooth structure without detrimental effect on pulp. The ablation per pulse is only 0.04-4 μm. ArF excimer laser produces a specific fluorescent light. This fluorescence spectrum allows checking the fluorescence of removed tissues, e.g., carious tissue, enamel, dentine, etc. If the spectrum differed from predefined limits of intensities, lasing is to be stopped. Er:YAG laser ablation of enamel/dentine can cause microscopic and macroscopic irregularities, which may offer a micro-retentive mechanism of adhesion without acid etching.

Er:YAG laser was used for the first time to prepare holes in the enamel and dentine in 1988. There were no cracks with little or no charring in the prepared cavity. For effective cutting, at least 1 mm of clearance is needed between the laser tip and tooth structure with 2–20 Hz frequency, 50–1000 mJ pulse energy and power 1–8 W depending upon the type of dental hard tissue.

Ajilal SK et al. (2012) compared the carious dentine excavated surfaces by tungsten carbide bur, Carisolve and Er,Cr:YSGG laser and found that lased carious dentine is scaly, irregular without smear layer.

5.4.2 *Laser Gingival Retraction* Argon laser is more absorbed by hemoglobin and hemosiderin. This characteristic is beneficial for retraction and hemostasis of the gingival tissue in preparation for crown and bridge. It is being attempted to fuse enamel along the prepared margins of abutment with laser which may prevent secondary caries as well as post-insertion sensitivity.

After tooth preparation, argon laser is used for hemostasis and retraction of gingival tissue. With the fiber of 300 μm, argon laser is inserted into the gingival sulcus in a sweeping motion which coagulates the small bleeding vessels and removes the sulcular linings and help for making a clean impression.

5.4.3 *Laser Etching* Acid etching of enamel is one of the important steps for composite resin restoration where strong acid like 30-50% orthophosphoric acid is being used. Laser was also tried to etch enamel/dentine. Initially CO_2 and Nd:YAG lasers were used with unsuccessful results.

Eversole and Rizoiu (1995) showed that etching of enamel and dentine by the erbium laser has been shown to be 'facilitated or even improved over acid etching techniques'. Visuri et al. (1996) showed that the bond strengths of lased dental surfaces had improved when compared to acid-etched and hand-piece controls.

Hadly (2000) had evaluated lased tooth surfaces for their ability to form adhesion with various bonding agents.

As per Convissar (2000), the laser etched enamel showed similar micro-retentive pattern comparable to acid-etched enamel.

Krishnan KV et al. (2013) compared the shear bond strength of orthodontic brackets etched with Er:Cr:YSGG and 37% phosphoric acid etching and concluded that laser with 2W/20 Hz produced adequate bond strength which could be an alternative to conventional etching.

5.4.4 *Laser Photo Polymerization* Argon laser at 488 nm visible blue wave length activates the photo initiator of composite resin and causes polymerization. The power output of 250-500 mW is usually used with 10 second single pulse with 5 mm spot size. It will produce a power density of 1.25-250 W/cm^2 which can cure up to a depth of 2 mm. Argon lasers can be used for curing composite resins which in turn are used for various purposes like fractured incisal edge, conservative class II, class III, and class V lesions.

Photo polymerization of light cured glass ionomer, calcium hydroxide base/liners and dentine bonding agents can also be done with argon laser. Time required to polymerize and access to the areas are the drawbacks of conventional light cure system which is overcome by argon laser with wide variety of fiber sizes for reduction of polymerization time.

5.5.5 *Laser Desensitization* Laser can be used to eliminate dentinal hypersensitivity effectively. But the exact mechanism of action is not very clear. GaAlA laser is thought to act by blocking the neural transmission and dentinal fluid movement. Er:YAG laser is used more effectively to treat dentinal hypersensitivity.

5.5.6 *Restoration Removal* Laser can also be used to remove dental cements, composite resin and glass ionomer cement but it should not be attempted to remove amalgam, cast and ceramic restoration. Because there is potential release of mercury in amalgam restoration and low absorption of other materials with reflection of the laser light, removal of aforesaid materials should not be tried.

5.5.7 *Application in CAD-CAM System* To develop a moiré pattern in CAD-CAM, a three dimensional solid-state laser based imaging is used to scan the prepared tooth for restoration/fixed partial denture to create computer file with data. To determine accurate surface wear of enamel and restorative materials, optical contour mapping of occlusal surface is done with laser.

5.5.8 *Bleaching* Bleaching light source is one of the most important factors for success of thermocatalytic bleaching. The light source can be of halogen, plasma arc, or light-emitting diodes (LED). Carbon dioxide laser, diode, Nd:YAG,Er:YAG and argon ion laser can also be used as a source of bleaching light. The wavelength may range from high ultraviolet spectra, low visible blue light spectra, to invisible infrared spectra such as that of CO_2 laser. Laser absorption enhancing particles are added in laser bleaching gel which contains chemophores or an activator that is specific to the wavelength of the laser. Although there is no added advantages of using laser lights for bleaching it is supposed to enhance the bleaching efficacy by activating the bleaching gel, either through a specific catalyst or through heat, to promote the decomposition process of hydrogen peroxide. Due to potential hard and soft tissue damage by CO_2 laser, American Dental Association council on scientific affairs has not recommended its use.

APPLICATIONS OF LASER IN THE FIELD OF ENDODONTICS

The following are the applications of laser in Endodontics

5.6 DIAGNOSTIC

1. For Assessing the Vitality of Pulp

The most appropriate way to check the vitality of pulp is by assessing the pulpal blood circulation. Laser Doppler Flowmetry (LDF) is the accurate way to assess pulpal blood flow, which will give the exact pulpal status.

Holloway GA and Walkins DW did the first application of LDF in medicine in 1977 for measuring blood flow of retina.

It was Gazelius et al (1986) who first studied the role of LDF to differentiate vital and non-vital pulps in humans. They also assessed the pulpal blood flow of four luxated mandibular central incisors of an 11-year-old boy after 1 week, 6 weeks, 9 months and 1 year following trauma.

Kim et al first convinced and confirmed that LDF assessed pulpal blood flow when they compared pulpal blood flow in dog canine teeth by LDF and 133-xenon wash-out methods.

Although LDF is the most accurate method to assess pulp vitality, it has certain drawbacks like:

- High setup cost
- The probe is very sensitive to movements
- Stabilizing stent should be prepared for each patient
- Position of the dental chair should be the same while recording

Principle When photons hit stationary tissue cells, they scatter without shifting their frequency, however when they hit moving blood cells, they scatter with shifting the light frequency according to Doppler principle.

Procedure

- Prior to placement of the stent, the gingival should be covered with aluminum foil or preferably with a dark rubber band.
- As body position affects the reading, the patient should be in a similar position in the dental chair.
- A stabilizing stent have to be fabricated with the help of rubber base impression material for each patient individually. This will help to reduce the artificial movements as well as the tooth will always be tested in the same location of the crown.

Uses

- It can be a useful adjunct for luxated teeth showing early signs of unfavourable outcome.
- It can predict the teeth at risk early after trauma.
- It can detect revascularization following replantation of avulsed tooth.

5.7 PREVENTIVE PURPOSE

5.7.1 Preventive Endodontics

Traditional way of doing indirect/direct pulp capping is by application of therapeutic materials like calcium hydroxide and MTA (mineral trioxide aggregate) which will encourage the formation of reparative dentine. But it requires considerable amount of time. The dentinal tubules can be sealed by Nd:YAG and 9.6 μm CO_2 laser. CO_2 laser (9.6 μm) causes ablation, melting and re-solidification of hydroxyapatite of enamel and dentine. Use of Nd:YAG laser with an energy below 1 W, 10 Hz with 10 sec. exposure time did not significantly elevate intrapulpal temperature.

As the remaining dentine thickness is lesser, therefore lower laser parameter should be used. Hemostatic effect of CO_2 laser on exposed pulp tissues of dogs is well appreciated by Melcer et al (1987). Success rates of CO_2 laser pulp capping was showed to be superior by Moritz et al (1998).

TREATMENT

5.7.2 During Treatment Phase

Different lasers can be used during different phases of endodontic treatment.

1. **Pulpotomy** Clinical success rate of 97% and radiographic success rate of 94% was achieved by Liu (2006) when he used Nd:YAG laser on human primary molar for pulpotomy.

2. **Sterilization/disinfection of root canals** One of the triad of success of endodontic treatment is "Microbial control" which can be achieved by use of proper irrigants and intracanal medicaments with wide spectrum of activity with shaping of the root canals. However, many endodontic pathogens like *Enterococcus faecalis, Provotella endodontalis,* etc., are resistant to routine protocols due to factors like limited antibacterial spectrums, failure to diffuse into the dentinal tubules.

There had been attempts to use lasers for root canal disinfection. CO_2 and Nd:YAG lasers were used first for disinfection of root canals and found to disinfect the dentinal tubules. Some other studies that used XeCl, Er:YAG, KTP-Nd: YAG, diode, Er:YSGG, Nd:YAP, Er,Cr:YAG and argon lasers for root canal disinfection and smear layer removal showed favourable results.

Bergman et al in their *ex vivo* study on effect of Nd:YAG laser on endodontic pathogens concluded that it is a possible supplement but not an alternative to existing protocol for root canal disinfection.

As the laser beam is emitted straight, it is impossible to clear the lateral walls of root canals. Therefore improvement of the endodontic tip is recommended by Matsumoto et al. (2000) in laser in endodontics.

In 1997 US, FDA had approved Er:YAG laser for use on dental hard tissues which gave popularity of laser amongst the clinicians.

Stabholz et al. (2003) developed a new endodontic tip for use along with Er:YAG laser system. Here, the beam of Er:YAG laser is delivered through a hollow tube with an endodontic tip having side firing activity which allows lateral emission of the irradiation suitable for lateral wall of the canal. The end point of endodontic tip is sealed so that it will help to prevent transmission of irradiation through the apical foramen. They studied the efficiency of this new tip on removing debris and smear layer from palatal root canals of freshly extracted human molars.

Delivery system used for endodontic application are either by a hollow tube (CO_2 and Er:YAG) or by thin optical fiber (Nd:YAG, KTP–Nd:YAG, Fr; YSGG, diode and argon). These systems have the potential to kill endodontic pathogens.

5.7.3 Photodynamic Therapy (PDT)

One of the drawbacks of routine cleaning and shaping in endodontic therapy is its inability to eliminate the endodontic pathogens resulting in failures. This is most often due to bacteria resistant to routine antimicrobial irrigants and agents. *E. faecalis, Streptococcus intermedius, Provotella endodontalis* are some of the examples. PDT was attempted for such organisms.

Seal et al. (2002) used PDT against *Streptococcus intermedius* biofilm and found it to be not equally effective as 3% sodium hypochlorite which may be due to improper delivery of the laser light. However, it may be a useful adjunct in reducing bacterial load in achieving resolution of periapical periodontitis.

Soukos et al. (1998) also concluded that methylene blue-sensitized *E. faecalis* when exposed to laser of 222 J/cm^2 energy density eliminated 97% of the organism from the experimentally infected root canal.

Garcez et al. (2008), Pinheiro et al also showed similar reduction of endodontic pathogen which further encourage us to use PDT in eliminating endodontic pathogens from root canals.

5.7.4 Root Canal Preparation

Liesenhoff T attempted *in vitro* as well as *in vivo* root canal preparation with excimer laser (308 nm) and found it to be successful.

5.7.5 Obturation

The final step of root canal treatment is obturating the prepared root canal with an inert material. Traditionally, gutta-percha (a transpoly isoprene of rubber) is used for obturation. Resin-based obturating material resilon (epiphany system) can also be used for obturation. Argon 488 nm laser was used to polymerize a resin used for obturation.

There is significant improvement of apical seal when Nd:YAG laser was used.

Er:YAG laser enhanced the adhesion of epoxy resin based sealers when compared with zinc oxide eugenol based sealers.

5.7.6 Endodontic Retreatment

Nd:YAG laser (1, 2 & 3 W) output was used to remove gutta-percha and broken instruments from root canals by Yu et al. (2000). They removed GP in 70% of the samples and removed broken files in 55% samples.

The time required to remove any obturating materials by laser was significantly shorter than conventional method. Use of lasers like Nd:YAG and Er:YAG are definitely advantageous which will eliminate the use of toxic solvents.

5.7.7 Apical Surgery

Miserendino used CO_2 laser during apical surgery to eradicate the apex. Improved hemostasis, potential sterilizing effect of contaminated root apex, root dentin permeability reduction, recrystallization of the root dentine are some of the added advantages of CO_2 laser apicoectomy.

Ebihara et al used Er:YAG laser for retrograde cavity preparation. Karlovic et al found that Er:YAG laser-prepared root end cavity showed lower microleakage irrespective of retrograde materials. Stabhold et al also used Er:YAG for apicoectomy with clean resected surface devoid of charring.

Gouw-Soares et al had given a protocol for laser apical surgery. Er:YAG can be used for osteotomy and root resection whereas Nd:YAG can reduce bacterial contamination of surgical cavity. However, LILT Ga-Al-As diode laser gives better healing potential with no adverse signs and symptoms.

5.7.8 Instrument Sterilization

Laser can also be used to sterilize endodontic instruments. Adrion J.C. first used CO_2 laser for sterilization of endodontic instruments.

T.W. Hooks et al found 100% of the spores were killed by CO_2 laser in contaminated endodontic instruments.

Powel G.L. and Whisenant B.K. (1991) studied the effectiveness of three lasers (Argon, CO_2 and Nd: YAG) to sterilize dental instruments. Of the three lasers tested, argon laser was capable of sterilizing selected dental instruments at lowest energy level (1 watt for 120 sec.). The other two lasers were able to sterilize instruments also, but at higher energy levels. Results indicated that all lasers were capable of sterilizing selected dental instruments; however the argon was able to consistently sterilize at the lower energy level of 1 watt for 120 sec.

5.8 LOW LEVEL LASER THERAPY (LLLT)

It is also known as "cold", "soft", "biostimulation" or photobiostimulation where laser with low energy density of visible red or near infra red spectrum of light is used. It has been used to alleviate pain after extraction, in post-herpetic neuralgia, aphthous stomatitis, TMJ dysfunction syndrome, trigeminal neuralgia and other chronic orofacial pain. It is also used to enhance healing, in TMJ arthritis, etc. The analgesic and other effects are due to decreased C-fiber activity, altered pain threshold and increased synthesis of bradykinins and endorphins.

Asnaashari. M., Mohebi. S., and Paymanpou. P. (2011) had used LLLT to reduce the pain after endodontic surgery and got encouraging results.

This type of laser unit is usually a small hand-held or bench-top model which is of low cost, not requiring integral cooling mechanism like surgical laser. Usually diode laser, argon laser and CO_2 laser had been used for low level laser therapy.

Laser of low energy density is used in the following purposes mentioned in the earlier parts of this chapter like photopolymerization of composite resin, for early detection of caries, in photodynamic therapy (PDT) and in CAD-CAM dentistry for scanning the prepared tooth/teeth or to study the wearing pattern of teeth.

With the advent of new dental tissue friendly laser systems, better understanding of the laser–tissue interactions, advancement in the laser delivery system, strict laser safety and patient's awareness for drill-free dentistry, time is not far to get the dental practice free of dental drills with lasers.

References

1. Einstein A. 1916. *Verk Deutch Phys Ges*. 18:318

2. Maiman T.H. 1960. Stimulated optical radiation in ruby. *Nature*. 187:493-494.

3. American Medical Association, Council of Scientific Affairs. Lasers in medicine and surgery. *JAMA*. 1986; 256:900-910.

4. Leo J Miserendino. 1995. History and development of Laser Dentistry: In *Lasers in Dentistry*. Leo J Miserendino, Robert M Pick, Quintessence Publishing Co. Inc., Singapore.

5. Goldman L. 1991. Background to laser medicine - History, principles and safety. In Goldman (ed): *Laser Non-surgical Medicine*. Lancaster, PA Technomic Publishing Co. Inc.

6. http://www.photonics.com/LinearCharts/Default.aspx?ChartID=2

7. Bjelkagen H, Sunderstrom F, Angmar-Mansson B et al. 1982. Early detection of enamel caries by luminescence excited by visible laser light. *Swed Dent J*. 6:1-7.

8. Kutsch V.K. 1992. Caries illumination with the argon laser: a clinical trial. *ISLD Third International Congress on Lasers in Dentistry*. p22.

9. Hibst R and Gall R. 1998. Development of diode laser based fluorescence caries detector. *Caries Res*. 32:294

10. Loben R.R and Fine S. 1966. Interaction of CO_2 laser radiation with oral hard tissues. *J Prosthet Dent*. 16:589.

11. Kantola S. 1972. Laser induced effects on tooth structure. *Acta Odontol Scand.* 30:463-484.

12. Stewart L, Powel G.L, and Wright S. 1985. Hydroxyapatite attached by laser: a potential sealant for pits and fissures. *Oper Dent.* 10:2-5.

13. Nelson D.G.A., Shariati M., Glena R., Cheilds C.P. and Featherstone J.D.B. 1986. Effect of pulsed low energy laser irradiation on artificial caries like lesion formation. *Caries Res.* 20:289-299.

14. Stabhold A, Kettering J, Neev Joseph, and Torabinejad M. 1993. Effect of Excimer laser on *Streptococcus mutans*. *J endod.* 19(5):232-235.

15. Satoaru O, Yuichi Y, and Minoru T. 1995. *In vitro* study of the effect of lasers irradiation on *Streptococcus mutans*. In *Lasers in Dentistry*. Leo J Miserendino, Robert M Pick, Quintessence Publishing Co. Inc., Singapore. p247.

16. Leo J Miserendino. 1995. History and development of Laser Dentistry: In *Lasers in Dentistry*. Leo J Miserendino, Robert M Pick, Quintessence Publishing Co. Inc., Singapore, p17

17. Natália Costa Araújo, Carla Raquel Fontana, Vanderlei Salvador Bagnato, and Marleny Elizabeth Martinez Gerbi. 2012. *Photo medicine and Laser Surgery*. 30(7): 393-399. July 2012

18. Meyers T.D, Meyers W.D. 1985. The use of the laser for debridement of incipient caries. *J Prosthet Dent.* 53:776-779.

19. Koort J Frentzen M. 1989. Excimer laser: Basic physics and possible applications in dental surgery :In *Lasers in Dentistry*. Yamamoto H, Atsumi K, Kusakari Haruka *Excerpta Medica*, Elsevier Science Publishers B.V. Amsterdam, p138

20. Margolis F.S. 2009. *Private Dentistry*. May 2009. 14-22

21. Ajilal S.K, Sam R.J.E, Babu R, and Suganthan P. 2012. Morphological changes in the caries excavated dentin prepared by Rotary, Carisolve™ and Er,Cr:YSGG Laser (Biolase™) instruments: A Scanning Electron Microscopic evaluation. *Int. J Laser Dent.* 2(1):1-6

22. Kutsch V.K and Blankenau R.J. 1995. Surgical applications of the Argon Laser In *Lasers in Dentistry*. Leo J Miserendino, Robert M Pick, Quintessence Publishing Co. Inc., Singapore. p133

23. Eversole L.R and Rizoiu I.M. 1995. Preliminary investigations on utility of an erbium, chromium, YSGG laser. *CDA journal.* 41-47, Dec.1995

24. Visuri, S.R., et al. 1996. Shear Strength of composite bonded to Er:YAG laser-prepared dentin. *J Dent Res.* **75**: 1, 599-605

25. Hadley, J. et al. 2000. A Laser-Powered Hydrokinetic System. *JADA*; **131**:777-785,

26. Convissar R.A. 2000. The Dental Clinics of North America. Philadelphia, WB Saunders

27. Krishnan K.V, Kumaran N.K, Iyer V.H and Rajasigamani K. 2013. Laser etched Vs Conventional etched enamel: Effect on shear bond strength of orthodontic brackets. *Int. J Laser Dent.* 3(1):1-6

28. Blankenau R, Kelsey W.P, Kutsch V.K. 1995. Clinical applications of argon laser in restorative dentistry. In *Lasers in Dentistry*. Leo J Miserendino, Robert M Pick, Quintessence Publishing Co. Inc., Singapore. p217-230.

29. Schwarz F, Arweiler N, Georg T, and Reich E. 2002. Desensitizing effects of Er:YAG laser on hypersensitive dentine: a controlled, prospective clinical study. *J Clin Periodontology*. 29:211-15

30. Dostalova T, Jelinkova H, Krejsa O, Hammal K , Kbelka J, et al. 1998. Er:YAG laser ablation: Clinical evaluation. *J Clin Laser Med Surg.* 16(5):273-82.

31. Dang M, and Shetty O. Nine shade change with laser-assisted tooth whitening. 2013. *Int. J Laser Dent*. 3(2):73-76

32. American Dental association council on scientific affairs: Report on laser bleaching. 1998. *J Am Dent assoc.* 129 (10) : 1484

33. Sigurdsson A. 2008. Laser doppler flowmetry In Ingle's *Endodontics*. Ingle J.I, Bakland L.K, Baumgartner J.C. CBS Publishers & Distributors Pvt Ltd. Indian edition for BC Decker Inc. p 547.

34. Gazelius B, Olgart L, Edwall B, Edwall. 1986. Non invasive recording of blood flow in human dental pulp. *Endod Dent Traumatol.* 2:219-21.

35. Kim S, Liu M, Markowitz K, et al. 1990. Comparison of pulpal blood flow in dog canine determined by the laser Doppler and the 133 xenon washout methods. *Arch Oral Biol.* 35:411-43

36. White J.M, Fagan M.C and Goodis H.E. 1994. Intrapulpal temperatures during pulsed Nd:YAG laser treatment, *in vitro*. *J periodontal.* 65:255-9

37. Melcer J, Chaumate M.T, and Melcer F, et al. 1985. Preliminary report of the effect of CO_2 laser beam on the dental pulp of the *Macaca mulatta* primate and the beagle dog. *J Endod.* 11:1-5.

38. Moritz A, Schoop U, Goharkhay K. 1998. The CO_2 laser as an aid in direct pulp capping. *J Endod.* 24:248-51

39. Jeng-fen Liu. 2006. Effects of Nd: YAG laser pulpotomy on human primary molars. *J Endod.* 32:404-7.

40. Bergman L, Moisiadis P, Teughel W, et al. 2006. Bactericidal effect of Nd:YAG laser irradiation on some endodontic pathogens *ex vivo*. *Int Endodo J.* 39:547

41. Matsumoto K. 2000. Lasers in endodontics. *Dent. Clin of North Am.* 44:889-906.

42. Stabholz A, Zeltzser R, Sela M, et al. 2003. The use of lasers in dentistry: principles of operation and clinical applications. *Compend.* 24:811-906.

43. Seal G.J, Ng Y.L, Spratt D, Bhatti M, Gulabivala K. 2002. An *in vitro* comparison of the bactericidal efficacy of lethal photosensitization or sodium hypochlorite irrigation on *Streptococcus intermedius* biofilms in root canals. *Int Endod J.* 35(3):268–274.

44. Soukos N.S, Ximenez-Fyvie L.A, Hamblin M.R, Socransky S.S, Hasan T. 1998. Targeted antimicrobial photochemotherapy. Antimicrob Agents Chemother. 42(10):2595–2601.

45. Garcez A.S, Silvia Cristina Nuñez, Michael R. Hamblin, P and Martha Simões Ribeiro. 2008. Antimicrobial effect of photodynamic therapy on necrotic pulp and periapical lesion. *J Endod*. 2008 February; 34(2): 138–142.

46. Pinheiro E.T, Gomes B.P, Drucker D.B, Zaia A.A, Ferraz C.C, Souza-Filho F.J. 2004. Antimicrobial susceptibility of *Enterococcus faecalis* isolated from canals of root filled teeth with periapical lesions. *Int Endod J*. 37(11):756–763.

47. Liesenhoff T. 1995. Clinical and investigative Research on the excimer Laser In *Lasers in Dentistry*. Leo J Miserendino, Robert M Pick, Quintessence Publishing Co. Inc., Singapore. p176-183

48. Pots T.V and Petrou A. 1990. Laser photo polymerization of dental materials with potential endodontic applications. *J Endod*. 16:265-8.

49. Gekelman D, Prokopowitsch I, Eduardo C.P. 1999. *In vitro* study of the effects of Nd:YAG laser irradiation on the apical sealing of endodontic fillings performed with and without dentin plugs. *J Clin Laser Med Surg*. 17: 261-6.

50. Yu D.G, Kimura Y, Tomita Y, et al. 2000. Study on removal effects of filling materials and broken files from root canals using pulsed Nd:YAG laser. *J Clin Laser Med Surg*. 18:23-8.

51. Miserendino L.L. 1988. The laser apicoectomy: endodontic application of CO_2 laser for periapical surgery. *Oral Surg Oral Med Oral Pathol Oral Radiol Endod*. 66: 615-9.

52. Ebihara A, Wadachi, Sekine Y, et al. 1998. Application of Er:YAG laser to retrograde cavity preparation. *J Japan Soci Laser Dent*. 9:23-31

53. Karlovic Z, Perelj-Ribaric S, Miletic I, et al. Er-YAG laser versus ultrasonic in preparation of root-end cavities. *J Endod*. 31:821-3.

54. Stabhold A, Zeltzser R, Sele M, et al. 2003. The use of lasers in dentistry: principles of operation and clinical applications. *Compend*. 24:811-24

55. Gouw-Soares S Stabhol A, Large-Marques L.J, et al. 2004. Comparative study of dentine permeability after apicectomy and surface treatment with 9.6 micrometer TEA CO_2 and Er:YAG laser irradiation. *J Clin Laser Med Surg.* 22:129-39.

56. Gouw-Soares S, Tanji E, Haypek P et al. 2001. The use of Er: YAG, Nd:YAG and Ga-Al-As. Lasers in periapical surgery: a three year clinical study. *J Clin Laser Med Surg.* 19: 193-8.

57. Adrian J.C and Gross A. 1979. A new method of sterilization: the carbon dioxide laser. *J Oral Path and Med.* 8(1):60-61.

58. Hooks T.W, Adrian J.C, Gross A, and Bernier W.E. 1980. Use of the carbon dioxide laser in sterilization of endodontic reamers. *Oral Surg Oral Med Oral Pathol.* 1980 Mar; 49(3):263-5. .(Abstract)

59. G. Lynn Powell and Brian K. Whisenant B.S. 1991. Comparison of three lasers for dental instrument sterilization. *Laser surgery medicine.* 11(1) 69-71.(Abstract)

60. Parker S. Low-level laser use in dentistry.*BDJ*; 202(3) 131-138.

61. Asnaashari M, Mohebi S, and Paymanpou P. 2011. Pain Reduction Using Low Level Laser Irradiation in Single-Visit Endodontic Treatment. *J Lasers in Med Sciences*; Vol 2, No 4. (Abstract)

6

Laser Applications in Prosthodontics

Dr. R. Shakila & Dr. L. Jeevanandam

Department of Prosthodontics,

Mahatma Gandhi Postgraduate Institute of Dental Sciences,

Indira Nagar, Puducherry

Prosthodontics is the area of dentistry pertaining to the diagnosis, treatment planning, rehabilitation, and maintenance of the oral function, aesthetics, and health of patients with clinical conditions associated with missing teeth, deficient teeth, and/or compromised maxillo-facial tissues using biocompatible substitutes. Prosthodontics involves a number of disciplines that include the following:

I) Complete denture prosthodontics

i) Prototyping and CAD/CAM (Computer Aided Design and Computer Aided Manufacturing) technology

ii) Analysis of occlusion by CAD/CAM

iii) Analysis of accuracy of impression by laser scanner

II) Fixed partial denture

i) Tissue management

ii) To treat dentinal hypersensitivity

iii) Pretreatment of non-precious alloys

iv) Crown preparation

III) Removable partial denture

Laser welding

IV) Implant dentistry

i) Soft tissue surgery

ii) Implant surface debridement

iii) Implant surface treatment

V) Maxillofacial prosthodontics

i) Sintering with CAD/CAM technology

6.1 COMPLETE DENTURE PROSTHODONTICS

6.1.1 Prototyping and CAD/CAM Technology

The term rapid prototyping (RP) refers to a class of technologies that can automatically construct physical models from Computer-Aided Design (CAD) data. These "three dimensional printers" allow designers to quickly create tangible prototypes of their designs, rather than just two-dimensional pictures. Such models have numerous data.

In addition to prototypes, RP techniques can also be used to make tooling (referred to as rapid tooling) and even production-quality parts (rapid manufacturing). A software package slices the CAD model into a number of thin (e.g., 0.1 mm) layers, which are then built up one atop another. Rapid prototyping is an additive process, combining layers of paper, wax, or plastic to create a solid object.

In contrast, most machining processes (milling, drilling, grinding, etc.) are "subtractive" processes that remove material from a solid block. RP's additive nature allows it to create objects with complicated internal features that cannot be manufactured by other means.

6.1.2 Laser Rapid Forming of a Complete Titanium Denture Base Plate

This technique uses the combination of the CAD/CAM and LRF (Laser Rapid Forming) methods for forming the titanium plate of a complete denture. Laser scanner, reverse engineering software, and standard triangulation language (STL) formatted denture base plate and sliced into a sequence of numerical controlled codes.

The denture plate will be built layer-by-layer, on the LRF system. After the traditional finishing techniques, this denture plate will be acceptable for use in patients.

6.1.3 Study of Complete Denture Occlusion using Three-Dimensional Technique

After fabrication of new dentures, the occlusion can be examined and studied with the help of laser scanner technique and three-dimensional reconstruction. The relationship between the parameters of balanced occlusion can also be analyzed.

6.1.4 Analysis of Accuracy of Impression by Laser Scanner

Several studies have made comparisons in the dimensional accuracy of different elastomeric impression materials. Most have used two dimensional measuring devices, which neglect to account for the dimensional changes that exist along a three-dimensional surface.

The scanning laser three-dimensional (3D) digitizer can delineate x, y, and z coordinates from a specimen without actually contacting the surface. The digitizer automatically tracks coordinates with precision and stores data as the number of points on a surface with a resolution of 130 mm at 100 mm. These exacting features suggest that the laser digitizer might accurately and reliably measure the dimensions of dental impression materials while avoiding subjective errors.

The image is built up and landmarks identified which allow superimposition of the images and so enable the differences between two similar images to be calculated.

The 3D laser captures complex 3D texture-mapped models and they are exported into a 3D (Scan Surf) software application where it is built and triangulated into a 3D meshwork image of the object. The scanning process is accomplished within a minute whereas the software analysis takes much longer. The software superimposes the two objects by either registering landmarks or by registering as iterative closest point (ICP). This finds an optimal fit between the two surfaces and in effect acts as a reference area. Once superimposed, the difference of the two surfaces is calculated as the shortest distance of each point on one object surface from a second object surface, within a range of 0.5 mm.

Three-dimensional digitizers will eventually become less expensive, require less maintenance, track faster, and be available with more standardized software.

6.2 FIXED PARTIAL DENTURE

6.2.1 Tissue Management

Crown Lengthening This is a procedure when inadequate crown height is present for crown restoration. An adequate crown height is created by removing required gingival soft tissue.

With the help of the lasers, soft tissue crown lengthening can be done without raising a flap. By its thermal effect, the laser seals vascular and lymphatic vessels; at the same time it vaporizes the excessive gingival tissue.

Since no flap was required for this surgery, sutures were not necessary and the wound healed by secondary intention.

Advantages

- Increased coagulation that yields a dry surgical field and better visualization.
- Tissue surface sterilization and therefore, reduction in bacteremia.
- Decreased swelling and edema of target tissue.
- Decreased pain, and in some cases no need of anesthesia while surgery.
- Faster healing response and increased patient acceptance.
- Less chair-side time.

6.2.2 To Treat Dentinal Hypersensitivity

There are many theories to describe the mechanism of hypersensitivity, but all conclude that open dentinal tubules are the path of stimuli to elicit response.

The first laser use for the treatment of dentine hypersensitivity was reported by Matsumoto et al (1985) using Nd:YAG laser. Many of the lasers investigated can induce significant thermal effects, if laser parameters are inadequately controlled, giving rise to concerns regarding thermal damage to temperature-sensitive pulpal tissue.

6.2.2.1 *Mechanism of Action of Lasers in Treating Dentinal Hypersensitivity* The precise mechanism of the ablation of hard tissues with the laser remains unclear. One theory suggested that when laser interacts with the hard tissue it is absorbed by the water and hydroxyapatite. The laser heats the water causing it to become steam. This expansion during the change of state of water causes cracking of the tissue. As the steam expands, it also forces the cracked material away from the ablation zone. Because this is a very rapid action, it is explosive (micro explosion) in nature. The lasers used for the treatment of the dentinal hypersensitivity are of the following types:

i) He-Ne Laser

The first use of this laser for the treatment of dentine hypersensitivity was reported by Senda et al. (1985). Irradiation modes were of two types: pulsed (5 Hz only) and continuous wave (CW) mode. Treatment effectively ranged from 5.2 to 100%.The mechanism involved is mostly unknown, but according to physiological experiments it increases the action potential of related nerve fibers. Its action will be long-lasting.

ii) GaAlAs Laser

The first use of this laser for the treatment of dentine hypersensitivity was reported by Matsumoto et al. (1985). An output power of 30 mW was used for the treatment. Irradiation mode was CW, and irradiation time ranged from 0.5 to 3 min. Treatment effectiveness ranged from 85 to 100%. The mechanism of action involved is blocking the depolarization of C-fiber afferents (Wakabayashi et al. 1992-1993).

iii) Nd: YAG Laser

The first use of this laser for the treatment of dentine hypersensitivity was reported by Matsumoto et al. (1985). The output power used may vary but 1-2 W is sufficient most commonly. The use of black ink as absorption enhancer is recommended when using Nd:YAG laser to prevent deep penetration of the laser beam through the enamel and dentin and excessive effects on pulp.

iv) CO_2 Laser

The first use of this laser for the treatment of dentine hypersensitivity was reported by Moritz et al. (1996). Effect of this laser on dentinal hypersensitivity treatment is due to the occlusion or narrowing of dentinal tubules. This laser irradiation may also cause dentinal desiccation; yielding temporary clinical relief of dentinal hypersensitivity (Fayad et al.1996). CO_2 laser with 1 W for 5-10 s duration could treat dentin hypersensitivity without adversely affecting the pulp.

v) Er:YAG Laser

This laser came up after all the above to avoid some of the disadvantages they have. These lasers are basically advantageous than above in the nature that these produce very less heat while application due to better absorption by water and hydroxyapatite. Desensitizing effects of this lasers are effective and long-lasting compared to above lasers at 80 mJ and 3 Hz output. Its desensitizing effect is attributed to the deposition of insoluble salts in the exposed dentinal tubules.

vi) Er:Cr:YSGG Laser

This is a recent laser tool used in dentistry for a variety of purposes. The mechanism of dentin removal as explained above for other erbium lasers is by "thermo mechanical process" in which the emitted laser light is absorbed by the water within the hydroxyapatite of a dental hard tissue. The water is then heated and evaporated, resulting in a high pressure of steam that causes a micro explosion of tooth tissue below the melting point of tooth tissue (approximately 1,200°C). Cumhur Sipahi, Nukhet Berk and Julide Ozen (2006) showed that long time-low potency (LT/LP) Er,Cr:YSGG lasers at 0.5 W potency for 30s produce required dentinal tubule closure to treat dentinal hypersensitivity.

6.2.3 Crown Preparation

Crown preparation with lasers is a debated topic still. There are no conclusive studies on the use of lasers for crown preparation purposes. But still some commercial companies say that they can be used. The following are the details regarding what these companies say:

Er,Cr:YSGG laser is used most commonly now.

i. It uses hydrokinetic technology (laser-energized water to cut or ablate soft and hard tissue).

ii. Because of this mechanism, local anaesthesia is not required in many cases, making this a more comfortable procedure for the patient, and of course, saving time and anaesthetic use by the patient.

iii. The laser hand piece resembles a high-speed hand piece but with fiber-optic tips instead of a bur, which directs the laser energy at a focal point approximately 1-2 mm from the tissue surface.

The crown preparation should be started on maximum setting for cutting enamel (6 W, 90% air, 75% water), started with a defocused mode for 30 seconds to 1 min. for anaesthesia of tooth.

iv. While placing the gingival margin, setting will be reduced to 1.25 W, 50% air, 40% water to control the cutting tip, for the purpose of accuracy.

v. To finish with the interproximal, buccal, lingual/palatal, reduction cuts will be performed with the dentin settings 4 W, 65% air, 55% water.

vi. The laser has to be reset at 2.25 W, 65% air, 55% water to finish the buccal cusp overlay, and the final margination of the proximal and lingual surfaces.

Advantages For vital crown preparation, no need of local anaesthesia, as laser causes temporary paresthasia of nerve endings.

Procedure is accurate and faster than the conventional method.

Disadvantages Trained dentists are required.

Crown Lengthening

Clinical scenarios where crown lengthening procedures are indicated within aesthetic zone require special consideration to achieve predictable aesthetic results. Crown lengthening procedures with the help of lasers are indicated in following conditions:

1. Caries at gingival margin
2. Cuspal fracture extending apical to the gingival margin
3. Endodontic perforations near alveolar crest
4. Insufficient clinical crown length
5. Difficulty in placement of finish line coronal to the biological width
6. Need to develop a ferrule

7. Unaesthetic gingival architecture

8. Cosmetic enhancements

Lasers offer unparallel precision and operator control and may be beneficial for finely tracing incision lines and sculpting the desired gingival margin outline. All the other crown lengthening procedures have certain disadvantages—as in surgical approach healing time is longer, post-healing gingival margin position is unpredictable, patient compliance is poor as it needs use of anaesthesia and scalpel for electro-surgery, and the heat liberated has a deleterious effect on pulp and bone leading to pulpal death or bone necrosis. Orthodontic extrusion leads to vertical bone defect adjacent to extruded tooth and it also needs patient compliance.

APPLICATIONS OF LASER IN CROWN LENGTHENING PROCEDURES

I. Soft Tissue Management Around Abutments

Argon laser energy has peak absorption in hemoglobin, thus lending itself to providing excellent haemostasis and efficient coagulation and vaporization of oral tissues. These characteristics are beneficial for retraction and haemostasis of the gingival tissue in preparation for an impression during a crown and bridge procedure. Argon laser with 300 um fiber, and a power setting of 1.0W, continuous wave delivery and the fiber is inserted into the sulcus in contact with the tissue. In a sweeping motion, the fiber is moved around the tooth. It is important to contact the fiber tip with the bleeding vessels. Provide suction and water spray in the field. Gingivoplasty may also be done using argon laser.

II. Modification of soft Tissue Around Laminates

The removal and re-contouring of gingival tissues around laminates can be easily accomplished with the argon laser. The laser can be used as a primary surgical instrument to remove excessive gingival tissue, whether diseased, secondary to drug therapy, or orthodontic treatment. The laser will remove tissue and provide haemostasis and tissues weld the wound.

III. Osseous Crown Lengthening

Like teeth mineralized matrix of bone consists mainly of hydroxyapatite. The water content and hydroxyapatite are responsible for the high absorption of the Er: YAG laser light in the bone. Er: YAG laser has very promising potential for bone ablation·

IV. Formation of Ovate Pontic Sites

There are many causes of unsuitable pontic site. Two of the most common causes are insufficient compression of alveolar plates after an extraction and non replacement of a fractured alveolar plate. Unsuitable pontic site results in unaesthetic and non self cleansing pontic design. For favorable pontic design re-contouring of soft and bony tissue may be needed. Soft tissue surgery may be performed with any of the soft tissue lasers and osseous surgery may be performed with erbium family of lasers.

V. Altered Passive Eruption Management

Lasers can be used very efficaciously to manage passive eruption problems. When the patients have clinical crowns that appear too short or when they have an uneven gingival line producing an uneven smile, excessive tissue can be easily and quickly removed without the need for blade incisions, flap reflection, or suturing.

VI. Laser Troughing

Lasers can be used to create a trough around a tooth before impression taking. This can entirely replace the need for retraction cord, electrocautery, and the use of haemostatic agents. The results are predictable, efficient, minimize impingement of epithelial attachment, cause less bleeding during the subsequent impression, reduce postoperative problems, and reduce chair time. It alters the biological width of gingiva. Nd:YAG laser is used. It vaporizes the epithelium which is attached to the marginal finish lines, the epithelium getting vaporized is only a transient loss and it forms again. After laser troughing the impression is taken and sent to the lab for prosthetic work. The most important function of marginal finish line is to maintain the biological width, it acts as the termination point of tooth preparation, help in ease of fabrication, helps in taking a proper impression. In brittle teeth to maintain the biological width and finish line laser troughing plays an important role.

6.3 REMOVABLE PARTIAL DENTURES

6.3.1 Laser Welding

Laser welding is one of the modern methods of removable partial dentures that uses the pulsed laser with relative low average power. This is known as a precise and rapid joining method, but its success depends on the control of many parameters,

e.g., for Co-Cr alloy frameworks.

The welding parameters were determined for each defect type and working step (fixing, joining, filling, and planning). Adequate combination of pulse energy (6–14 J), pulse duration (10–20 ms) and peak power (600–900 W) depending on the working stage improves the success of the welding procedure.

6.3.2 Removable Prosthetics

The successful construction of removable full and partial dentures mainly depends on the preoperative evaluation of the supporting hard and soft tissue structures and their proper preparation. Lasers may now be used to perform most pre-prosthetic surgeries. These procedures include hard and soft tissue tuberosity reduction, torus removal, and treatment of unsuitable residual ridges including undercut and irregularly resorbed ridges, treatment of unsupported soft tissues, and other hard and soft tissue abnormalities. Lasers also may be used to treat the problems of hyperplastic tissue and nicotinic stomatitis under the palate of a full or partial denture and ease the discomfort of epulis, denture stomatitis, and other problems associated with long term wear of ill-fitting dentures. Stability, retention, function, and aesthetics of removable prostheses may be enhanced by the following proper laser manipulations of the soft tissues and underlying osseous structure.

i. ***Treatment of Unsuitable Alveolar Ridges*** Alveolar resorption usually is uniform in vertical and lateral dimensions. On occasion, irregular resorption occurs in one of the dimensions, producing an unsuitable ridge. As the available denture bearing area is reduced, the load on the remaining tissue increases, which leads to an ill-fitting prosthesis, with discomfort that is not alleviated by soft linings[11] to remove sharp bony projections and to smooth the residual ridge soft tissue laser surgery to expose the bone may be performed with any number of soft tissue wavelengths (CO_2, diode, Nd:YAG). Hard tissue surgery may be performed with the erbium family of wavelengths.

ii. *Treatment of Undercut Alveolar Ridges* There are many causes of undercut alveolar ridges. Two of the most common causes are dilated tooth sockets that result from insufficient compression of the alveolar plates after an extraction and non-replacement of a fractured alveolar plate. Naturally occurring undercuts such as those found in the lower anterior alveolus or where a prominent pre-maxilla is present may be the cause of soft tissue trauma, ulceration, and pain when prosthesis is placed on such a ridge. Soft tissue surgery may be performed with any of the soft tissue lasers. Osseous surgery may be performed with the erbium family of lasers. During mastication, the upper denture oscillates, causing disproportionate resorption in the maxilla. The soft tissues are compressed, thus causing the denture to become increasingly unstable. Pain is not felt until the anterior nasal spine is nearly exposed and subject to trauma from the denture base. Unsupported maxillary alveolar soft tissues are bulkier than those in the lower jaw that tend to prolapse in the lingual direction. Traditional surgery consists of removing wedges of soft tissue from the alveolar crest until the wound edges are closed easily. Any of the soft tissue lasers are able to perform this procedure.

iii. *Treatment of Enlarged Tuberosity* The most common reason for enlarged tuberosity usually is soft tissue hyperplasia and alveolar hyperplasia accompanying the over-eruption of unopposed maxillary molar teeth. The enlarged tuberosity may prevent the posterior extension of the upper and lower dentures, thereby reducing their efficiency for mastication and their stability. The bulk of the hyperplastic tuberosity may lie toward the palate. Surplus soft tissue should be excised, allowing room for the denture bases. The soft tissue reduction may be performed with any of the soft tissue lasers. If undercuts are present, then osseus reduction may be required. Erbium laser is the laser of choice for the osseus reduction.

iv. *Surgical Treatment of Tori and Exostoses* Prosthetic problems may arise if maxillary tori or exostoses are large or irregular in shape. Tori and exostoses are formed mainly of compact bone. They may cause ulceration of oral mucosa. These bony protuberances also may interfere with lingual bars or flanges of mandibular prostheses. Soft tissue lasers may be used to expose the exostoses and erbium lasers may be used for the osseous reduction. A smooth, rounded, midline torus normally does not create a prosthetic problem because the palatal acrylic may be relieved or cut away to avoid the torus.

v. *Soft Tissue Lesions* Persistent trauma from a sharp denture flange or over compression of the posterior dam area may produce a fibrous tissue response. Hyperplastic fibrous tissue may be formed at the junction of the hard and soft palate as a reaction to constant trauma and irritation from the posterior dam area of the denture. The lesion may be excised with any of the soft tissue lasers and the tissue allowed re-epithelialization.

6.4 IMPLANT DENTISTRY

Dental lasers are used for a variety of procedures in implantology like implant recovery, implant site preparation and removal of diseased tissue around the implant.

i. Implant Recovery

Following the placement of implant and its integration into the osseous substrate, the current method of treatment is to surgically uncover the implant, wait for the tissue to heal, and then proceed with impressions and fabrication of the restoration. The reason for the delay is to facilitate the impression-taking process. Uses of lasers can greatly expedite this procedure because the implant can be uncovered and impressions can be obtained at the same appointment. All types of lasers can be used to expose dental implants. One advantage of use of lasers in implantology is that impressions can be taken immediately after second stage surgery because there is little blood contamination in the field due to the haemostatic effects of the lasers. There also is minimal tissue shrinkage after laser surgery, which assures that the tissue margins will remain at the same level after healing as they are immediately after surgery. In addition the use of laser can eliminate the trauma to the tissues of flap reflection and suture placement.

ii. Implant Site Preparation

Lasers can be used for the placement of mini implants especially in patients with potential bleeding problems, to provide essentially bloodless surgery in the bone.

iii. Removal of Diseased Tissue Around the Implant

Lasers can be used to repair ailing implants by decontaminating their surfaces with laser energy. Diode, CO_2 and Er:YAG lasers can be used for this purpose. Lasers can also be used to remove granulation tissue in case there is inflammation around an already osseointegrated implant.

Apart from the above mentioned uses implant dentistry has the following uses also:

i. For Sterilization of Socket

In immediate implant dentistry, after extraction of tooth, without any infection, socket can be sterilized immediately without any pain.

ii. In case of Peri-Implantitis

Since the laser does not transmit damaging heat, it can be utilized to vaporize any granulation tissue as well as clean the implant surface in peri-implantitis cases. This procedure eliminated the acute state of peri-implantitis, resulting in positive GTR (Guided Tissue Regeneration), and allowing the patient the extended use of the implant.

iii. To debride the implant surface

Miller Robert has shown that treatment of the contaminated implant surface by mechanical and chemotherapeutic means has met with mixed success. Development of a laser system operating at 2780 nm and using an ablative hydrokinetic process offers the possibility for more efficient decontamination and debridement. Laser ablation using the Er:Cr:YSGG laser is highly efficient at removing potential contaminants on the roughened implant surface while demonstrating no effects on the titanium substrate.

6.5 MAXILLOFACIAL PROSTHESIS

New advances in rapid prototyping technologies have demonstrated significant advantages compared to more conventional techniques for fabricating facial prosthesis. The use of selective laser sintering technology is an alternative approach for fabricating a wax pattern of maxillofacial prosthesis. This new approach can generate the wax pattern directly and reduce labour-intensive laboratory procedures.

6.5.1 SLS (Selective Laser Sintering)

The SLS (Selective Laser Sintering) is a method of computer aided designing using mainly the laser. In this method, models are generated directly from 3-D computer data then converted to STL files, which are then sliced into thin layers (typically about 0.1 mm/0.004 inches) using the associated computer software. The laser sintering machine produces the models on a removable platform by applying incremental layers of the pattern material. For each layer, the machine lays down a film of powdered material with an accurate required thickness, again a fresh film of powder is laid down, and the next layer is melted with exposure to the laser source. This process continues, layer by layer, until the pattern is completed.

Advantages Manufacturer time is reduced.

More precision can be achieved.

6.6 LASER WELDING TECHNIQUE IN PROSTHODONTICS

Since 1990, pulsed Nd-Yag dental lasers have been commercially used in Europe. Manufacturers present the laser welding technique as a new, rapid, economic and accurate way for joining metal. In prosthetic dentistry, this technique has the following advantages:

- The laser device saves time in a commercial laboratory because all welding is done directly on the master cast. Inaccuracies in assembly caused by transfers from the master cast along with investment and heat distortions are reduced.

- It is consistently possible to weld very close to acrylic resin or ceramic parts with no physical (cracking) or colour damage.
- Potentially, all metals can be joined but particularly titanium alloys.
- Laser welding joints have a high reproducible strength for all metals, consistent with that of the substrate alloy.

Considering all these advantages, all dental technician should have a laser in their laboratory. However, looking at the available literature, since 1970 many experiments have been conducted using non-precious and precious alloys and have shown contradictory results, probably because the experimental procedures used were different. Therefore no comparison could be made. In this experiment, the weldability of three non-precious alloys was investigated. The procedure consisted of determining the appropriate welding parameters which could achieve a deep joining in depth without cracks or gas entrapments in the welding area. The quality of the joining was checked by metallographic observations on polished sections. Wires of different diameters were then laser-welded and tested in tension. In order to understand the different behaviours between the three alloys (2 Ni-Cr and 1 Co-Cr based alloys), the composition of the welded area was determined by x-ray microprobe. Particular attention was given to the role played by the impurities.

6.6.1 Laser Parameters and Welding Conditions

In order to determine the welding conditions against the metal thickness and the ability of the laser device, two series of cast wires (0.6 to 2 mm thick), and five specimen DIN 50125 (3 mm thick) were prepared by investment casting. The samples were then cut, joined by hand, edge to edge and welded without fillers or fluxes, using a commercial Nd-YAG laser (DL 2002 manufactured by Dentaurumm). In order to avoid the laser beam reflection and to improve the weld penetration, all the wires were sand-blasted with alumina powders and welded under argon shielding atmosphere to decrease the oxidation contamination.

6.7 LASER APPLICATION IN DENTAL LABORATORY

There is a range of laboratory-based laser applications. Laser holographic imaging is a well established method for storing topographic information, such as crown preparations, occlusal tables, and facial forms. The use of two laser beams allows more complex surface detail to be mapped using interferometry, while conventional diffraction gratings and interference patterns are used to generate holograms and contour profiles. Laser scanning of casts can be linked to computerized milling equipment for fabrication of restorations from porcelain and other materials. An alternative fabrication strategy is to sinter ceramic materials, to create a solid restoration from a powder of alumina or hydroxyapatite. The same approach can be used to form complex shapes from dental wax and other materials which can be sintered, such that these can then be used in conventional 'lost wax' casting. A variation on this theme is ultraviolet (helium-cadmium) laser-initiated polymerization of liquid resin in a chamber, to create surgical templates for implant surgery and major reconstructive oral surgery. These templates can be coupled with laser-based positioning systems for complex reconstructive and orthognathic surgical procedures.

7

Laser Safety in Dentistry

Prof. Dr. S. Mohan

Vel Tech University, Chennai 600 062

7.1 INTRODUCTION

Laser is a wonderful and unique radiation. Even now only few doctors and nurses in our country know what a laser is and fewer use it in ophthalmology, dentistry and ENT. Shortly lasers are going to be a standard tool in our medical and surgical wards. Hence one has to learn to manage this exciting dynamic technology.

Traditional medical service, whether in a hospital or private practice requires a wide range of technical and administrative skills to employ lasers. When lasers are introduced, the skills have to be modified with a new knowledge based on biophysics, high-tech instrumentation and safety. Although lasers are not new to medical field, it has taken quite a long time to gain widespread acceptance. Recently, lasers are rapidly accepted in medical practices, dental, surgery and at treatment centers.

In the last several years, technological changes have made a variety of lasers available in health care. With the increased use of lasers and multiple wavelengths in medicinal fields like dentistry and surgery, laser safety requires specific guidelines. This demands an urgent need for doctors and nurses to learn about lasers. The inclusion of a laser to patient's treatment plan takes considerable doctor's time in addition to their responsibility to educate, counsel patients and to provide physical and emotional support.

It is essential for dentists working with lasers to have an understanding of the fundamentals of the technology and its integration into current practice. In the earlier chapters, we have already discussed about lasers in dentistry in general and prosthodontics and conservative dentistry and endodontics in particular along with basic laser physics, tissue interaction and different types of lasers. To know, more about laser uses, one has to look at an important question, viz., how do we protect the dental team (i.e., the dentist, assistant) and the patient from laser radiation? Since lasers are considered as a high risk source, all health care personal who work with lasers should be well acquainted to biophysics and laser safety.

7.2 LASER DELIVERY SYSTEMS

All lasers regardless of their properties and biophysical effects can cut, coagulate and vapourise tissue to some degree. The wavelength determines the typical delivery system to be used. Carbon dioxide laser energy must be delivered by means of hollow tubular system with mirrors to reflect the beam down to the output device.

Methods of delivering carbon dioxide laser radiation include hand pieces, microscope adaptors, rigid endoscopes and both flexible and semi-rigid waveguides. All other wavelengths can be transmitted across fiber optics. Laser fibers and flexible quartz come with various coatings to protect the core and purge channels are created for coaxial cooling. Today's fibers are disposable, durable and reliable and come in a wide variety of sizes and configurations. Fibers make use of flexible endoscopes. It opens up new horizons where the areas unreachable with either the carbon dioxide laser or conventional instrumentation, can be reached with this technology.

Contact tips and sculptured fibers are used in contact with the tissue and deliver a thermal effect. This technique converts the Nd: YAG laser from a coagulation device to a device that can cut and coagulate simultaneously.

Regardless of the delivery system, the dental use of laser energy requires a focusing device to produce a small spot of energy that can be carefully and controllably directed to the operative site. Focusing lenses built into the delivery system (hand piece, fiber and microscope connector, etc.) can be short or long, allowing the beam to focus at varying distance from the tissue. As the distance from tissue changes, so does the size of the laser beam. That is, when the beam is focused to a very small spot, the energy is concentrated into a high power density beam which cuts or vapourizes tissue rapidly and precisely. As the beam moves away from tissue, the spot size increases and lowers energy concentration so that with low power density, only a shallow surface effect is created.

Irradiation time affects the depth of penetration and hence we should take care of tissue damage. Time exposure is usually measured in terms of joules or watts multiplied by time. The total dosimetry is expressed in terms of energy density (Watts × time × area or spot size). This determines the complete picture of tissue effect regardless of wavelength.

7.3 LASER SAFETY SYSTEMS

The lasers always have in-built safety systems such as emergency 'Stop' button, shutters to prevent laser emission in the absence of proper delivery system , foot-switch to avoid accidental operation, control panel, visual signs of laser emission, locked unit to prevent unauthorized tampering of laser parts, password protection and remote inter-locks.

Before admitting the patients to the dental chair, the dentist or the laser safety officer should test-fire the laser to confirm that the laser is working correctly. Laser control measures are:

1. Power or energy output.
2. Pulse length.
3. Pulse repetition rate.
4. Wavelength.

5. Beam path.

6. Beam shape.

7. Number of laser systems at a particular location.

8. Laboratory layouts, position of windows, doors, etc.

9. Degree of isolation of location.

10. Type of population (informed staff in control, local knowledgeable personnel, and uninformed personnel).

7.4 LASER HAZARDS

A laser can be considered as a high source of extremely intense electromagnetic radiation that is defined by three basic characteristics, viz., monochromatic, directional and coherent. Due to the temporal and spatial coherence of the laser beam, it can be considered as a point source with the brightness exceeding that of sun. Lasers are a more directional light source than any other radiation. The higher the optical output powers of the laser, the greater the potential hazard.

The hazards from lasers can be divided into five categories:

1. Eye hazards such as retinal or cornea burns,

2. Skin hazards such as burns,

3. Electrical hazards from high voltage equipment,

4. Fire hazards, and

5. Laser plume.

Eye hazard is the major hazard from laser radiation which enters the eye since eye is the most sensitive organ to light. The lens in the human eye focuses the laser beam into a tiny spot that can burn the retina. The visible and near infrared range of the spectrum have the greatest potential for retinal injury, as the cornea and lens are transparent to these wavelengths and the lens can thus focus the laser energy onto the retina. The maximum transmission by the cornea and lens, and the maximum absorption of laser energy in the retina falls in the range from 550 nm to 400 nm. Argon and YAG lasers emit radiation in this range and hence they are the most hazardous lasers. Wavelengths of less than 550 nm can cause a photochemical injury similar to sunburn. Photochemical effects are cumulative and result from exposures of over 10 seconds to diffuse or scattered light. When a laser beam enters the human eye retinal burns can occur. Laser beams are almost parallel thus the lens of the human eye will focus them down to a small spot. A laser beam with low divergence entering the eye can be focused down to a spot 10 to 20 microns in diameter. The energy density (energy per unit of area) of the laser beam increases as the spot size decreases. That is, the energy of a laser beam can be intensified up to 100,000 times by the focusing action of the eye. A one watt laser beam when focused down to a small spot can produce temperatures higher than the surface temperature of the sun. Thus even a low power laser in the mill watt range can cause a burn if focused directly onto the retina.

Skin hazard is the exposure of the skin to high power laser beams (1 or more watts) which can cause burns. The heat from the laser beam under five watt levels will cause a flinch reaction before any serious damage occurs. The sensation is similar to touching any hot object. With higher power lasers, a burn can occur even though the flinch reaction may rapidly pull the affected skin out of the beam. These burns can be quite painful as the affected skin is burnt and forms a hard lesion that takes ages to heal. UV lasers are not used in dentistry, as it can cause ablative damage to skin and may lead to pre-cancerous state.

Electrical hazards are due to the laser operating voltage. Most medium and high power lasers operate on 220 or even higher AC voltages which draw lots of current and frequently use multi-phase electrical connections. The power supply (exciter) for the laser typically doubles or even triples the line voltages before feeding them to the laser head where lethal voltages can be present. An additional electrical hazard exists where water cooling of the power supply (exciter) is used. Minor leaks in the water cooling pipes can cause high voltages to short to the water or case of the unit both of which are usually at ground potential.

Fire hazards occur unexpectedly while using lasers. High power laser beams deflected onto flammable materials can cause ignition and fires. A 10 watt laser will drill a hole in cinder block when focused. Almost any material except metal is a potential fire hazard, especially wood and drapes. Nylon or rayon clothing is especially bad for burns as the plastic fabric melts and can cling to skin increasing the burn duration and intensity. Hose connections at the water feed and the hoses themselves can leak. Water cooling system can also leak in unexpected places inside the equipment causing flooding and water damage. When working around laser, it is best to wear shoes that have insulated soles.

Laser plume

Laser plume arises due to the laser tissue ablation. Whenever noncalcified tissue is ablated, such as in caries removal and all soft tissue surgeries, water vapour, hydrocarbon gases, carbon monoxide and dioxide and particulate organic material (including bacteria and viral bodies) are emitted. The effect of plume inhalation can be serious and cause nausea, breathing difficulties and distant inoculation of bacteria.

7.4.1 SAFETY PRECAUTIONS

Eye Safety—Laser safety glasses/goggles with specially coated lenses should be used. The coatings on the lenses are designed to absorb or attenuate certain wavelengths so that if one is accidentally struck in the eye by the beam, damage is minimized. Unfortunately these glasses often make it difficult if not impossible to see the beam. A pair of welders' goggles will work as they reduce the light to the eyes by a factor of 10X to 50X. While welding goggles will not give total protection, they may reduce the beam power down to levels where damage is less likely. (Stay outside of any 'safe zone' around lasers at shows. The 'safe zone' is there to prevent audience's access to the laser equipment and to prevent spectators from harming themselves or being hit by laser beams).

Electrical Safety—One should follow the same kinds of safety precautions around lasers as with any other power tool or electrical device.

Sign Boards—In laser operating areas, sign boards such as 'Caution: Laser in Use' or 'Danger Laser Radiation' should always be used. This sign contains an area at the bottom where the details of the laser type (Argon Laser) and output power (100 mW) are inscribed.

7.5 LASER HAZARD CLASSIFICATIONS

The classification of laser hazards is based upon the intensity of the emitted beam. It describes the ability of the laser to injure personnel.

Essentially all of the dental lasers (those that by definition are used to vaporize or burn tissues) are classified as class 4 lasers. Commonly used dental lasers are argon laser (488-514 nm), Diode lasers (810-980 nm), Nd:YAG (1064 nm), Ho:YAG (2100 nm), Er,Cr:YSGG (2780 nm), Er:YAG (2490 nm) and CO_2 laser (10600 nm). These lasers present potential burn hazards from even diffuse reflections of the beam, if close enough to the reflecting surface. The lower classes of lasers present potential eye hazards, varying in chance and severity with the class of hazard.

Class 1 laser These lasers are exempt from general controls because they present no hazards when used under ordinary circumstances. These include lasers like small semiconductor gallium-arsenide (GaAs) lasers (810-890 nm) used in low level light therapy.

Class 2a lasers These are very low power visible lasers which will not present hazards, even if viewed directly, for short periods of time. They are not intended for prolonged viewing—in the range not to exceed 1000 seconds (over 15 minutes of direct viewing). Common experience will reveal that one cannot even stare directly into a 100 watt light bulb for that length of time without discomforting effects. This should put laser hazards into some perspective.

Class 2b lasers These are low power visible lasers which normally do not present a viewing hazard, but only because of the normal human aversion response. (Blinking and/or turning away within 0.25 seconds). They could present a problem if viewed for extended periods of time. It is interesting to note that this level of hazard also applies to many conventional light sources (like endoscopic light sources). They include low power lasers such as He-Ne laser pointers or the grocery store scanners (around 5 mW). The only way to be hurt is to intentionally overcome one's natural aversion and stare directly into the beam. (This is about as hard as intentionally staring into the sun).

Class 3a lasers These lasers are safe if viewed only momentarily with the unaided eye but the use of collecting optics may create the hazard.

Class 3b lasers These are lasers that can definitely produce a hazard when viewed directly, including the intrabeam viewing of specular reflections (acutely reflected beams such as from a mirror like surface). Only the higher powered 3b lasers present hazards from diffuse reflections.

Class 4 lasers These include most of the surgical laser systems, which produce hazards from both specular and diffuse reflections. They may also present fire and skin burn hazards.

The laser class, power and their corresponding hazards are summarised in the following table.

Table 7.1 Laser class, power and their corresponding hazards

Laser-class/ power	**Brief**	**Expo-sure**	**Long**	**Expo-sure**	**Due to specular reflec-tion**	**Expo-sure to skin**
	Magnified exposure	Without safety spectacles	Magnified exposure	Without safety spectacles		
1 /mW	No risk	No risk	No risk	No risk	No risk	No risk
2a /mW	No risk	No risk	High risk	High risk	No risk	No risk
2b	High risk	No risk	High risk	High risk	No risk	No risk
3a / W	Take precaution	Take precaution	High risk	High risk	No risk	No risk

3b	High risk	High risk	High risk	High risk	Take precaution	Take precaution
4 / high power	High risk	High risk	High risk	High risk	High risk	High risk

7.6 SAFETY MEASURES

When laser light falls on the tissue, scattering occurs below the surface of the tissue (forward scatter) or of the tissue surface (backscatter). Each wavelength creates different amounts of scattering, with different consequences.

Carbon dioxide laser has no backscatter because it is absorbed immediately in the surface water, allowing visibility of each plane of tissue as vaporization occurs. This controls depths and prevents deep tissue damage leading to scarring and other complications.

Nd:YAG produces deep forward scattering radiation and a large amount of backscattering. As the portion of the laser beam scattered off the surface of the tissue, the energy efficiency creates an ocular hazard which requires careful monitoring and protective lenses.

Visible laser usually penetrates not more than 3 mm but do produce backscattering. But Nd: YAG laser wavelength react to light colored tissues due to increased backscattering. Darker tissues with large amounts of pigments or vasculature reduce backscattering due to increasing absorption. This can lead to unwanted tissue damage and scarring. Surface areas adjacent to the operative site must be protected to avoid this complication when using a laser such as argon or KTP laser.

Reflection can occur whenever a laser beam strikes a specular surface. Even though the intensity of the energy may be decreased in the reflected beam, it is still a hazard. Black instruments can still be reflective, if they do not have a dull or roughened surface to diffuse the energy. All instruments to be used in the direct path of the laser beam should be anodized to prevent reflection hazards.

The high energy of the laser and the potential for promoting combustion pose special problems when the surgical field is in close proximity to the airway. An endotracheal tube can be converted into flaming blowtorch with catastrophic injury to the patient. To minimize the incidence of such complications, anesthesiologists who are involved in laser airway surgery should be familiar with the elements of laser operation, the type of lasers and special anesthetic considerations for safe laser surgery.

Laser dental/surgery hazards can be broadly classified as follows:

	Operation Theatre/ Dental chair	**Human**
a) Fire	a) Fire	a) UV, plasma, free radical generation
b) Electric shock	b) Smoke	b) Shock wave, heat and light
	c) Environmental gas pollution	c) Dentist
	d) Explosion of anesthetic agent	

Unless safety measures are followed completely (without compromise), the use of laser energy to both patient and personnel are not safe.

In USA, the American National Institute (ANSI) document z-136.3 is the only nationally accepted, non-regulatory guideline for laser safety. This document is increasingly referenced by regulatory agencies, the military, professional organizations, and institutional accreditation agencies.

The Australian/New Zealand Standard 4173:1994 serves as the national guidelines in those countries and is used as the guideline for some Pacific Rim countries as well. This document was published in 1994 and is comprehensive and understandable.

Some issues addressed in most standards include administrative control or laser services (laser committee, polices/procedures), the role and responsibility of the laser safety officer, hazard identification, control measures, selection of eyewear, airborne contaminants, terminology, service and testing and an appendix of recommendations for many surgical specialties.

Before a laser is used clinically, a program should be established according to standards and guided by written polices and procedures, documentation forms and appropriate quality management systems.

Though the revised ANSI standard is no longer mandatory, a laser committee can serve to monitor an institution's safety program. Representation should include hospital administration, laser safety officer, operating room supervisor, biomedical engineer, continuing education managers, physicians from each specialty, anesthesia, marketing and risk management. Meetings should be scheduled frequently during the first year of a new laser program. A physician is usually appointed to chair the committee, with the laser safety officer appointed as co-chair. Agenda items can include education, technology assessment, new applications, equipment acquisition, documentation and statistics review, marketing, budget, policy updates, and expansion strategies.

The Laser Safety Officer (LSO) or laser scientist or laser engineer supervises the clinical, technical and administrative components of the laser program. The position may be filled by a laser trained personnel, biomedical engineer or other properly trained person who will be available in the operating theatre whenever lasers are in use. The LSO must have both responsibility and authority to monitor and enforce compliance with standards and policies. In hospital having minimal laser usage, the LSO can be a laser trained staff nurse or laser trained nursing supervisor with other duties. However, in large programs having multiple laser systems and multiple users, it is necessary for this position to be dedicated.

Some of the LSO's responsibilities include hazard evaluation and control of all laser systems and rooms, implementation of policies and procedures, education and training of staff, documentation review, laser committee functions, audits of safety equipment, evaluation of new instrumentation, revision of policies, patient education, marketing, research and supporting the laser team.

Dentist education should be complete for the development of safe practices in the operating room or at dental chair. By providing continuing education for physicians which includes updating specific characteristics and safety of new wavelengths, the laser safety can be greatly improved. Lasers are considered high-risk equipment. Education of all persons involved with laser utilization is of the utmost importance to prevent accidental injuries.

Educational programs for dentists, post graduates, undergraduates, technicians and supporting staffs at dental colleges should be taught by recognized experts in the field from the credible institution. Attendance during such a course should be required prior to practice. Validation through written exams, completion of skills, check list and demonstrations should be a component of every certification policy. An annual in-service is usually required in order to keep the staff in line with the current developments.

In multi wavelength hospitals, an increased potential for error can occur. For example, the different eye wears with different lasers becomes important. Violation can lead to inadequate protection for the safety. As the laser numbers increases wih several wavelengths, non-compliance commonly creeps in hospitals. Hence, the institution can colour code eyewear, provide a pocket resource for personnel and implement continuous quality improvement activities in order to improve safety practices.

Some laser procedure (patient under general anesthesia, high acuity extensive instrumentation, new operators, etc.) requires a third person staffed as the designated laser operator. This person can be a nurse, technician, biomedical or other properly trained person. The responsibilities of a laser operator are to set-up, test, operate and to repair troubleshooting laser equipment, monitor safety, document procedures and to communicate with the LSO.

When a local or regional anesthetic is used, it may be unnecessary to staff a third person. Patient safety, physician preference and staff skill level, may help the LSO to determine whether or not to assign a dedicated operator.

The baseline examination is usually required for all personnel who may have access to a laser treatment room, prior to beginning work with lasers.

Safety is everyone's responsibility. Dentists operating with laser must be familiar with the hospital policies and insist on compliance by all personnel in dental room.

Very strict safety is necessary for high intensity laser and its potential for tissue damage and combustion. The laser should not be aimed at highly polished or mirror-like surfaces. Tracheal laceration leading to late complications, tooth damage, injury to soft tissue and continuous burns to operating room personnel have been reported during laser surgery. The eye can be easily damaged by the laser and careful protection is mandatory. Unless safety measures are followed completely (without compromise), the use of laser energy to both patient and personnel are not safe. The carbon dioxide laser is absorbed by ordinary eyeglasses and hence adequate protection should be provided. The use of eyeglasses with side guards is suggested. Special glasses or goggles are required for all other lasers. In surgical theatres, the appropriate laser and an opaque covering of the operating room windows should be used. A warning sign should be placed on the operating room door to alert personnel to the use of the laser. A smoke evacuator should be used to eliminate the products of combustion. The patient should be draped with wet towels that are periodically moistened to keep them wet. Disposable operating room drapes can be flammable and difficult to extinguish since they are water repellent.

Patient safety depends on knowledgeable personnel and consistent application of known safety practices. Should anyone refuse to comply, an incident report should be written and a report made to the laser committee.

The LSO has the authority to evaluate an incident of non-compliance, and make a decision to either terminate or continue a laser procedure. This decision is usually based on several factors.

Laser hazards can also be divided into two categories, viz., beam hazards and flame hazards.

Beam hazards include flammability, reflection, skin burns, and ocular damage. These hazards are present whenever the laser is activated. For this reason, the laser operator should always be at the control of laser when it is in the operate mode and should always place the laser in the standby mode (disabling the shutter) when the beam is not focused on the target. It is important to keep the entire path of the beam free of obstruction and watch the operative site for interference.

Flammability hazards represent most of the accidents occurring with lasers. Dry disposable materials such as cotton, gauze, tongue blades, drapes, lap sponges and towels can ignite when a laser beam strikes. To prevent fire, place only wet materials in the operative field and remove all excess draping from the impact site. An open basin of water should be kept near the laser operator in case of fire in the surgical field. A fire extinguisher should be in the room or immediately available, in case of equipment fire. If non-woven drapes are used, a fire blanket should be in the room, to smother the material if such a fire occurs, since water cannot be used.

Another hazardous material is alcohol. Any compound or solution containing alcohol (including Hibitane, tape removers, skin degreasers and benzoin, etc.) can ignite if it comes in contact with the heat from the laser beam. Flash fires can also occur if the indoors in pooled or aerosolized betadine are heated by a focused laser beam. Nurses should evaluate each case for sterile, clean status and for potential risk to the patient and prepare the patient accordingly.

Whenever external areas of tissue are being vaporized with a carbon dioxide laser, a layer of carbon can build up. If carbon is allowed to remain, the beam will overheat it, causing extensive tissue damage, resulting in carbon sparking. If this occurs at the surface of the skin, it can cause fire, skin burns and injury to the surgeon. When this condition develops, stop lasing, irrigate the operative site and remove the carbon layer from the surface.

Biophysics explains that each wavelength interacts differently with tissue and therefore can produce different types of ocular injuries. Carbon dioxide absorbed in water will cause a corneal or surface burn of the eye, but depending on power density, the burns can go as deeply as 7-9 microns. Nd: YAG, KTP, and dye wavelengths can pass through water, clear structures, and are refocused by the human lens and strike the retina, causing damage to central vision.

Ocular damage is entirely preventable by wearing appropriate safety eyewear whenever a laser is in use. All eyewear is labeled with optical density and wavelength of protection afforded and it is essential that each individual read the labels before putting on protective eyewear, assuring that it is the correct pair.

Safety eyewear should be worn by all personnel in the room, when the laser is in the operative mode. Eyewear must be used during endoscopy or video procedures because of the potential for fiber breakage or mechanical accident, releasing uncontrolled and often invisible laser energy into the room. Wavelength specific safety lenses or filters are available for endoscope and microscopes and must be used over the viewing port to protect the surgeon.

Patients should receive the same eye protection as personnel, if they are awake during the procedure. Be sure the goggles fit properly and do not slide away when the patient lies down or changes position. For patients under general anesthesia, a wet cloth towel can be draped over the eyes for protection. Never use oil-based eye lubricant, dry eye pads, metal or plastic masks, to cover patient's eyes. Safety goggles can be placed over the eyes, if they can be held in place easily and safely and do not interface with anesthesia.

Optical density can be calculated by the LSO, according to published formulas for maximum permissible exposure or can be set at a level not less than 4.5 for most lasers in the clinical setting.

Non-beam hazards include mechanical accident, electrical hazards, failure to maintain controlled access and exposure to laser plume. Crowded operating rooms full of tangled power cords and with poorly positioned equipments are the leading causes of mechanical "laser" accidents. Equipments should be positioned away from doorways and the number of cords minimized. The footswitch should be given only to the credentialed laser surgeon, separated from all other pedal operated devices, to avoid mistaken activation of laser.

The laser is a high voltage electrical device and appropriate electrical safety precautions should always be taken. The laser operator should be sure that inflammable solutions and containers of fluids are not placed near lasers and all cords, footswitches, and circuit breakers should be checked periodically. Only properly trained and approved service technicians should be allowed to work on a laser, to remove the outside covers and to handle the electrical components.

Controlled access is the responsibility of the laser operator. Doors to a laser room should be cooled whenever the laser is in use and posted with "DANGER" signs. Safety goggles should be hung on the door sign, for the protection of anyone entering during laser operation. Signs should be removed when the laser is not in use.

Only those who are trained in laser safety should be allowed in the room when the laser is in use. Risk for accident increases when a room is crowded with people who do not understand the potential hazards.

All windows must be covered with shades or other filters, to prevent accidental transmission of a beam through the windows. Only the carbon dioxide beam is blocked by glass or plastic windows alone and therefore does not require additional window coverings.

The most effective way of limiting access to the laser is to keep the key in a secured place, allowing access only to those who are authorized to operate the equipment.

Laser-generated airborne contaminants are the subject of widespread debate. Research has shown that when human cells are heated to the point of disruption through the application of laser or electro surgical devices, the cellular content ejected contains harmful particulates, including DNA carbonaceous carcinogens and viral strands.

7.6.1 MANAGEMENT OF AN AIRWAY FIRE

The possibility of a fire in the airway during laser surgery makes it necessary that a plan of action be developed before this catastrophe occurs (Table 1). The endotracheal tube used should be secured with a minimal amount of tape so that easy extubation can be readily accomplished. Saline should be available to douse any flames. At the first sign of an airway fire, the anesthesiologist should stop all ventilation and terminate the flow of all anesthetic gases, including oxygen, since they promote combustion. After extinguishing any flames, the endotracheal tube should be quickly removed, since even brief combustion will damage the tube, making it unsuitable as an airway. The patient should be ventilated with a mask and the airway should be thoroughly examined. If the fire is quickly extinguished, little or no damage may occur. In such a case, the decision can be made to proceed with surgery. Extensive airway burns may necessitate mechanical ventilation, positive and expiratory pressure, antibiotics and steroids.

The Venturi jet ventilation technique was devised by Sanders as a means of artificial ventilation without the presence of an endotracheal tube. A catheter was clamped inside an operating bronchoscope or laryngoscope and was connected to a source of oxygen at 50 lb-per-square-inch pressure. With the use of a toggle switch, a jet of oxygen was directed down the bronchoscope. The result was adequate ventilation of an anesthetized patient. Using this technique, room air is entrained with the oxygen jet. When used with an operating laryngoscope, laser surgery of the vocal cords can be accomplished even in the posterior or interarytenoid areas normally obscured by the endotracheal tube. The absence of an endotracheal tube makes laser surgery easy and this technique produces no fire in the airway. The adequacy of ventilation and oxygen delivery by this technique has been demonstrated by measurement of arterial blood gas tensions. These steps should be taken simultaneously by the anesthesiologist and surgeon.

Table 7.2 Airway Fire Protocol

Cease ventilation and turn off all anesthetic gases including oxygen.
Extinguish flames with saline.
Remove endotracheal tube.
Ventilate by mask.
Evaluate airway for burns.

Pure oxygen is generally administered during jet ventilation because the entertainment of air will reduce the faction of oxygen that the patient receives. Inhalation anesthetics should be avoided, since they pollute the operating room. A totally intravenous anesthetic technique should be used.

Venturi jet ventilation uses a very high-pressure source in the airway. The 50-lb-square-inch pressure commonly used is equivalent to 3,500 cm water pressure. This is greatly in excess of normal airway pressures. These pressures may cause barotraumas such as pneumothorax or pneumomediastinum. No barrier to the passage of vomitus, blood, or debris into the trachea exists with this technique, since no cuffed endotracheal tube is used. The venturi jet must be kept in perfect alignment with the trachea or gastric dilatation with possible regurgitation may occur. An immobile field may be difficult to maintain because of the movement of the vocal cords by the jet.

The anesthesiologist should watch vigilantly for bilateral chest excursions to ensure adequate ventilation during jet ventilation. A precordial stethoscope should be used as well as the usual anesthetic monitoring devices described previously. The special endotracheal tubes such as Bivona "fome-cuff" nallinick-rodt, Xomed, and Norton laser endotracheal tubes are available at present.

Smoke evacuation systems are recommended for all plume producing procedures. Tubing should be held at no more than 2 cm from the impact site and instruments with collection ports may be necessary.

Wall suction can become clogged and lose its efficiency, if used without in-line filters placed between the wall and the suction canister. All filtration materials should be rated at levels of 0.1 micron or below, in order to remove known plume particulates.

Laser masks can provide added protection if worn properly. Plume cannot be filtered if it is drawn into gaps along the sides or under the nosepieces of tie-on masks. Laser masks should be worn during all plume producing procedures. It is important to remember to change laser masks after each case and discard them properly.

All plumes filtering equipment should be handled according to infection control procedures in the operating room. Used suction equipment is contaminated and universal precautions should be followed during handling and changing of tubing and filter canisters.

Safety education for patients helps to reduce their anxiety levels. Remember that protective eyewear limits eye contact and can interfere with patient–nurse communication. Prepare them ahead of time, by showing them photographs, perhaps bound in a brief booklet, demonstrating patients and staff wearing goggles, the equipment to be used and what a laser looks like as it strikes tissue.

Do not forget to show them a photo of the DANGER signs on the door and explain the reason for the warning. Seeing that sign on the way into the treatment room can scare the patient if they are not explained earlier.

Patients should be instructed to tell the nurse or doctor when they experience discomfort, so that the procedure can be managed without danger which may cause accidental burns. For laser safety, precaution, team work, and good communication are the most important.

Although we currently have lasers for use in virtually all surgical specialties, the future promises many exciting changes in the technology, as we move into the next century. Holographic imaging, virtual reality, minimally invasive instrumentation, tissue welding, biostimulation, multiwavelength systems, new wavelengths, diodes, and the dynamics of photobiology will change medicine and surgery in the near future.

Lasers and the professional members of clinical laser teams, partnered with industry, research centers, the government, and the international community, will make it all possible. Pre-operative nurses are vital members of these teams, with unlimited opportunities for new careers, professional growth and exciting challenges, as future technology becomes today's reality.

Nearly every laser currently used in medical applications is a class IV system and by definition they have potential for eye injury or fire hazard either by their direct or reflected beam. It is therefore necessary to identify these potential hazards and the various conditions that tend to influence these hazards in the normal use of laser energy. The regulations, hazards evaluation and analysis are an important part of laser curriculum. Thus, safety measures are at the most important in laser surgery and hence our nation needs more laser personnel, laser scientists and laser engineers.

Summarisingly,

1. As CO_2 ($\lambda = 10.6$ μm) lasers are frequently used in laser surgery, CO_2 laser goggles of 2 mm thick, optical density (O.D) - 0.35 can protect the eye.

2. Various types of burns develop according to direct or indirect (reflected) laser beam. Hence exposure to lasers should be avoided.

3. Non-inflammable and non-explosive anesthetic agents should be used.

4. For patients, non-flammable drape should be used. Non-operative field should be covered with normal saline soaked gauze. With intra oral lesion, appropriate care should be taken with orthodontic appliance and gold denture, etc.

5. All the shining operative instruments should be coated with black or chrome electrical coating.

6. Suction tip should be covered with rubber tube.

7. The operation table and other instruments in light should be non-reflecting, non-shining and heat tolerant.

8. Control of power is checked at the focusing head by calorimeter.

9. He-Ne (3 mW) should be used as light guide.

10. Lighting in the operation theatre should be proper.

11. The power of the laser for the operation of various organs depends on the size and the age of the person. The approximate power chart is as follows. The chart just gives an idea and the doctors are advised to start with low power from that mentioned in the chart.

Tissue	**Power**	**Tissue**	**Power**
Skin	5–15 W	Cartilage	15–20 W
Subcutaneous tissue	10–15 W	Bone	20–35 W
Fat	10–20 W	Kidney	25–35 W

Fascia	5–10 W	Liver	35–40 W
Muscle	10–20 W	Lung	25–35 W
Mucosa	5–10 W	Brain	20–35 W
		Peritoneum	5–10 W

Apart from power chart, the other factors to be kept in mind in performing laser surgery are:

1. At high power, tissue is cut more deeply.
2. With slow speed, the tissue is cut more deeply.
3. With low water content in the tissue, the cut is very deep.
4. With pressure, the cutting surface will separate more easily.

By keeping these points in mind, one can easily control the depth of cutting and can perform laser surgery safely.

Employees Responsibility

1. An employee shall not operate a laser without LSO's permissison.
2. Employees should obey the rules, regulations and procedures prescribed by LSO.
3. If there is any suspicion about the laser accident or the accident itself at the laser site, the employee should inform to the LSO immediately.
4. Whenever an employee is working with laser, he should use the safety equipment along with laser glasses and strictly follow the safety procedures.

Summarisingly, the control measures for laser hazards are the fiber optics tip must be steam sterilized in sterilizing pouches, use protective wear, use of screens, curtains and proper clothing, use of anti-fire explosive and project training and courses.

References

1. Scott E, Beswick A, and Wakefield K. 2004. The hazards of diathermy plume. Part 2. Producing quantifi ed data. *Br J Perioper Nurs*. **14:** 452, 454-456.

2. Garden J.M, O'Banion M.K, Bakus A.D, and Olson C. 2002. Viral disease transmitted by laser-generated plume (aerosol). *Arch Dermatol*. **138:** 1303-1307.

3. Kunachak S, and Sobhon P. 1998. The potential alveolar hazard of carbon dioxide laser-induced smoke. *J Med Assoc Thai*. **81:** 278-282.

4. McKinley I.B Jr, and Ludlow M.O. 1994. Hazards of laser smoke during endodontic therapy. *J Endod*. **20:** 558-559.

5. Laser Inst of America, Laser safety guide, 11th Edition, 2007

6. Association of peri-operative Registered Nurses Recommended Practices committee. Recommended Practices for laser safety in practice settings. 2004. *AORN.J.* 79, 836, 838, 841-44

7. Pioch T and Mattias J. 1998. *Eur J oral Sci*, , 106, 600-602

8. Jacques. A. 1989. *Nurs J*. 7, 5-9

9. Fisher.R.W. 1987. *Biomed. Technol*. Today. 191-194

10. Piccione. P.J. 2004. *Dent. Clin. North Am*. 48, 795-807

11. Toon.S. 1998. *Occup. Health Saf.* 57, 30

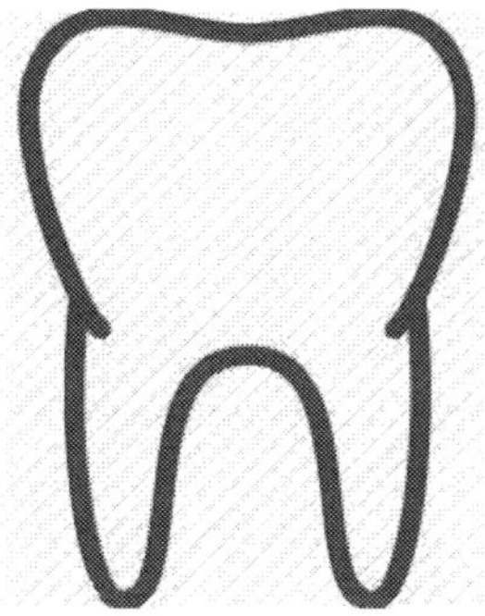

Glossary

Ablation The process of removing tissue with a laser through vaporization or mechanical disruption.

Active medium The laser component which produces laser light when stimulated. Dental lasers use crystals, gas, or semiconductors as their active media.

Abrasion Loss of tooth structure caused by a hard toothbrush or poor brushing technique.

Abscess A dental abscess may be caused by severe decay, trauma, or gum disease and will be characterized by swelling and pain. If an abscess ruptures, it can be accompanied by sudden relief from pain and a foul taste in the mouth.

Adhesive dentistry Term for dental restorations that involve "bonding" of composite resin or porcelain fillings to natural teeth.

Amalgam A silver/mercury mixture which is used for restoring lost tooth structure.

Anesthesia In dentistry we use local and general anesthesia. Numbing a tooth is an example of local anesthesia. Partial or complete unconsciousness is an example of general anesthesia.

Anterior teeth	The front six teeth, which are also referred to as incisors and cuspids.
Attrition	The loss of tooth structure due to wear.
Biopsy	The removal of a small piece of tissue for microscopic examination.
Bone graft	Surgical replacement of bone in preparation for a dental implant or to cosmetically replace missing bone.
Bonding	Adhering tooth-colored resin materials to restore the natural appearance of teeth. These materials can be sculpted and shaped to replace lost tooth structure due to decay or trauma and/or for cosmetic treatment.
Bridge	A fixed or removable dental appliance that replaces lost and/or missing teeth.
Chromophore	The tissue component that absorbs the laser energy and converts it into thermal energy.
Calculus	The scientific term for tartar, which is a hard deposit that typically forms due to poor oral hygiene. When plaque mineralizes and hardens it forms calculus. A hard deposit of mineralized substance adhering to crowns and/or roots of teeth or prosthetic devices.
Canal	The narrow chamber inside the root of the tooth that contains the nerve and blood vessels. Analogous to a wick inside a candle.
Canines	The third tooth from the center (cuspid).
Caries	Another name for a cavity (tooth decay).
Cavitron	A dental instrument that uses high frequency ultrasonic waves to remove calculus from teeth.

Cementum	A hard tissue that covers the root of a tooth.
Composite filling	Tooth colored restorations, also known as resin fillings that are typically completed in one sitting.
Composite resin	A tooth-colored material composed of plastic with small glass or ceramic particles that hardens either with a high intensity light or a chemical catalyst. A tooth colored resin combined with silica or porcelain and used as a restoration material.
Contouring	The process of reshaping teeth.
Cosmetic recontouring	A cosmetic procedure to shape the natural teeth to make them straighter or more youthful.
Cosmetic dentistry	The field of dentistry dedicated to the art and science of enhancing a person's smile, overall appearance and oral health.
Cracked tooth syndrome	When a tooth has a partial or complete fracture. Can be treated with a crown, root canal and/or extraction.
Crown	A restoration that covers all or part of a tooth, which typically requires two sittings. Crowns can be made of porcelain, gold, stainless steel, or composite. Also known as caps. This is also the portion of a tooth above the gumline. An artificial tooth replacement that restores missing tooth structure by surrounding the remaining coronal tooth structure. It is also placed on a dental implant.
Curettage	The act of removing infected tissue from a wound; used commonly in dentistry to refer to the removal of grossly inflamed gum tissue caused by periodontal disease.
Cusps	The highest point on the chewing surfaces of the back teeth (posterior teeth).
Cuspid (Canines)	The third tooth from the center of the mouth. These are part of the anterior group. Also known as a canine tooth.

Divergence	The tendency of the laser beam to spread outward once it exits the handpiece. Divergence varies depending on the specific laser and hardware used.
Decalcification	The loss of calcium from teeth. This weakens the teeth and makes them more susceptible to decay.
Decay	Destruction of tooth structure caused by toxins produced by bacteria.
Deciduous teeth	The first set of teeth a human is born with. Also known as baby teeth and primary teeth.
Dentin	The layer of tooth structure under the enamel. This layer is highly sensitive.
Dentition	The arrangement of natural or artificial teeth in the mouth.
Denture	A removable appliance that replaces all or some of the teeth. Can be an upper and/or lower prosthetic.
Diagnosis	The process of identifying the nature of a disorder, disease or condition.
Energy density	The amount of laser energy in an area of exposed tissue.
Er,Cr:YSGG	Erbium, Chromium-doped Yttrium Scandium Gallium Garnet crystal.
Er:YAG	Erbium-doped Yttrium Aluminium Garnet crystal.
Edentulous	When all of the teeth are missing from either the upper and/or lower jaw.
Enamel	The hard, white outer layer of the tooth that covers and protects the dentin.
Endodontics	The treatment of diseases and/or injuries that affect the root tip and/or pulp (nerve) of the tooth.
Endodontist	Specialist who treats injuries, diseases, and infections of the tooth pulp (nerve chamber).

Extraction The removal of a tooth.

Extrusion Tooth movement in the direction of eruption. The two types are mechanical extrusion—to move teeth with an applied force so that they extend farther out of the gums and natural extrusion—teeth naturally extrude from the bone until there is contact with another tooth.

Filling The restoration of lost tooth structure with tooth-colored or metal materials.

Fistula The channel emanating pus from an infection site. Also referred to as a gum boil.

Fluoride A natural element found commonly in nature in water, soil, air, and in a lot of foods. Fluoride is absorbed easily into the teeth's enamel to help protect the teeth from tooth-eating bacteria. It can be used as a topical such as in fluoridated toothpastes and gels or it can be absorbed systemically such as in fluoridated water, soft drinks, teas, and dietary supplements. The systemic fluoride that is retained by the body is absorbed by bones and teeth.

Fluorosis A harmless cosmetic discoloring of the enamel, which appears as chalky white specks and lines or pitted and brown stained enamel on teeth.

Fixed bridge A dental prosthetic used to replace missing tooth/teeth that is cemented or bonded to adjacent teeth, which have been prepared to provide the foundation for the prosthetic.

Forensic dentistry The gathering of legal evidence for identification or legal purposes.

Freeway space The distance between the upper and lower teeth with the lower jaw in rest position, which is typically the position immediately after swallowing.

Frenectomy	The removal or reshaping of thin muscle tissue that attaches the upper or lower lips to the gum, or the tongue to the floor of the mouth.
Frenum	Small pieces of pink colored skin that attach the lips, cheeks and tongue to the mouth. Examples include the piece of skin under the tongue, which sticks out when the tongue is lifted, and the piece of skin which sticks out when the lips are pulled out.
Genioplasty	Surgery of the chin, whereby its shape or size is altered.
General anesthesia	True general anesthesia is a deep state, and includes the loss of all reflexes and sometimes requires respiratory assistance. This state is rarely necessary for general dental procedures as all the most fearful patient wants is no pain, no consciousness of the procedures and no memory of the experience.
Gingiva	Gum tissue, which is pink and firm when it is healthy.
Gingival hypertrophy	The abnormal enlargement of the gingiva surrounding the teeth caused by poor oral hygiene or some medications.
Gingivectomy	The surgical removal of gum tissue.
Gingivitis	Inflammation of the gum tissue. Gingivitis is caused by the bacteria found in plaque that attack the gums. Symptoms of gingivitis include red, puffy gums and/or bleeding gums. When gingivitis is not treated, it can advance to periodontitis.
Gingivoplasty	The reshaping of gum contours, often for aesthetic purposes. Generally very easy and non-painful, it is often a good solution for a "gummy smile."
Gum disease	See gingivitis and periodontal disease.

Halitosis	Bad breath of oral or gastrointestinal origin.
Implant	Artificial tooth roots that are placed into bone to mimic the root structure of a tooth. They can be used to replace teeth or to support and retain dentures. A crown, bridge, or denture is then placed over the implant to restore natural tooth function.
Incision and Drainage (I and D)	A technique used to allow for the drainage of infections.
Incisor	The central or lateral front teeth with cutting edges. There are four upper (central and lateral) and four lower (central and lateral).
Impression	Mold made of the teeth and/or soft tissues. Impressions are used to make crowns, bridges, veneers, dentures, implants, some fillings, and study models.
Interproximal	The space between two teeth.
Intraoral	Inside the mouth.
Intrusion	Movement of a tooth back into the bone.
Keratin	A protein present in the organic matrix of the enamel of teeth.
Laser	Light Amplification by Stimulated Emission of Radiation
Labial	The tooth surface next to the lips. Usually refers to the front teeth.
Laminate veneer	A thin porcelain or composite resin facing that is bonded to teeth.
Local anesthesia	Relieves the sensation of pain in a specific area.

Mandible	The lower jaw.
Maxilla	The upper jaw.
Mechanical extrusion	To move teeth with an applied force so that they extend farther out of the gums.
Molars	The back teeth with the large chewing surfaces. They typically have from two to four roots and there are first, second and third molars.
milli Joule	Measurement of energy.
monochromatic	In laser science refers specifically to the fact that lasers produce a single wavelength of light.
Natural extrusion	Teeth naturally extrude from the bone until there is contact with another tooth.
Nd:YAG	Neodymium-doped Yttrium Aluminium Garnet crystal.
Optical pumping	Flash lamp stimulation of an active medium.
Output coupler	A semi-transparent mirror in the resonator that the laser beam passes through into the beam transfer hardware.
Occlusal	The chewing surfaces of back teeth.
Oral and maxillofacial surgeon	Orthopedic facial surgeon who is responsible for treating a wide variety of dental problems including the removal of impacted teeth (orthognathic surgery), abnormal growths, and reconstructive facial surgery.
Oral hygiene	The process of cleaning and maintaining the teeth and related structures.
Oral pathologist	Dentist specializing in the study of oral diseases.

Oral surgery	Surgery inside the mouth.
Oropharynx	The part of the throat at the back of the mouth.
Orthodontics	The dental specialty that focuses on the development, prevention, and correction of irregularities of the teeth, bite, and jaws.
Orthodontist	A dentist who has been specially trained in orthodontics.
Photobiomodulation	The process whereby laser energy is used to stimulate positive clinical outcomes such as pain relief and improved healing.
Power	Rate of doing work, measured in Watts.
Pulse duration	The amount of time a laser pulse is on, measured in microseconds.
Palate	Hard and soft tissue forming the roof of the mouth.
Palliative treatment	Non-invasive relief of irritating conditions.
Partial denture (bridge)	A removable appliance that replaces some of the teeth in either the upper or lower jaw.
Pedodontics	The area of dentistry that specializes in the treatment of children.
Pedodontist	A dentist who specializes in the treatment of children's teeth.
Periodontal disease (gum disease)	Inflammation of the bone and attached gum tissue. Clinically appears as loose teeth and/or bleeding gums. Can be treated non-surgically as well as surgically depending on the severity.

Periodontal maintenance	The periodic cleaning of the teeth, which usually follows periodontal treatment. Also known as a perio prophy or perio recall.
Permanent molars	The adult first, second and third molars that usually appear in six year increments starting at age 6.
Permanent teeth	The adult teeth.
Plaque	A film of bacteria that forms on the teeth and gums after eating foods that produce acids. If plaque is not removed, it hardens to form calculus or tartar, which can only be removed professionally.
Porcelain	A ceramic glass that fuses at high temperatures. This is used in crowns, bridges and veneers to mimic enamel.
Porcelain fused to metal (PFM)	Restoration with metal substructure that is covered with porcelain.
Porcelain inlay or onlay	A tooth-colored restoration made of porcelain, which is cemented or bonded in place.
Porcelain veneers	Ultra-thin, custom-made facings that are bonded to teeth to enhance and restore function and/or appearance. Veneers can be used to treat chipped, worn, crooked, and/or discolored teeth.
Post and core	Post and buildup to replace lost tooth structure for the purpose of retaining a crown.
Prognosis	The anticipated outcome of treatment.
Prophylaxis	The process of cleaning teeth, which is also known as a prophy.
Prosthesis	An artificial appliance for the replacement for a body part.
Prosthetics	A fixed or removable appliance to replace missing teeth. Fixed bridges, removable partials, and dentures are all examples.

Prosthodontics	The branch of dentistry concerned with the construction of artificial appliances designed to restore and maintain oral function by replacing missing teeth and sometimes other oral structures or parts of the face. Prosthodontics is one of the nine dental specialties recognized by the American Dental Association (ADA).
Prosthodontist	Dental specialist skilled in restoring or replacing teeth with fixed or removable prosthesis, maintaining proper occlusion; treats facial deformities with artificial prostheses such as eyes, ears, and noses.
Pulp	The inside part of the tooth that contains nerves, blood vessels and connective tissue. This is removed during a root canal procedure.
Pulp cap	Covering an exposed or nearly exposed nerve with a sedative material prior to restoring the tooth.
Pulpectomy	Complete removal of the pulp, which is commonly done in diseased children's teeth.
Radiograph	Another name for an X-ray.
Receding gums	A condition whereby the gums pull away from the tooth, which makes the tooth look longer since more of the tooth is exposed. This can be caused by buildup of plaque and/or poor brushing habits.
Resin-bonded bridge	A thin metal or glass fiber-reinforced bridge which usually requires slight modification of the adjacent teeth.
Restoration	Replacement of a portion of a damaged tooth.
Restorative	Procedures performed to restore the missing part of the teeth. Some insurance companies only consider fillings to be restorative; others consider fillings, crowns, bridges, and dentures to be restorative.

Root	Tooth structure that connects the tooth to the jaw.
Root canal	The common term for root canal therapy, which is also the interior space of the tooth root.
Root canal therapy	The nerve of the tooth is removed from the canal inside the root and replaced with a sterilized filling material.
Reflection	When the laser beam bounces off the surface with no penetration or interaction at all.
Resonator	The mirrored chamber surrounding the active medium that helps to amplify the laser light produced.
Saliva	Clear lubricating fluid in the mouth containing water, enzymes, bacteria, mucus, viruses, blood cells, and undigested food particles.
Salivary glands	Located under tongue and in the cheeks whose purpose is to produce saliva.
Scaling	Scraping of the teeth above the gums.
Soft palate	The muscular, movable part of the roof of the mouth.
Splint	Connection of two or more teeth so they function as a stronger single structure.
Stainless Steel Crowns	Silver colored crowns often used to restore heavily damaged baby molars and, occasionally, adult molars when a more long term crown is not an economic option.
Sterilization	A process where instruments are treated to remove all possible germs.
Scattering	The tendency of laser light to bounce in multiple directions once it enters tissue.
Stimulated emission	The process whereby the active medium is stimulated by an external source of light or electricity to produce laser light.

Tartar	Another name for calculus, which is the sticky film on teeth (plaque) that has hardened.
Tongue	A large muscle on the floor of the mouth that manipulates food for chewing and swallowing; the main organ of taste; assists in forming speech sounds.
Thermal relaxation	The ability of tissue to absorb and dissipate heat produced by pulsed dental lasers.
Transmission	When laser energy can pass through superficial tissues to interact with deeper areas.
Veneers (porcelain or composite)	Ultra-thin, custom-made facings bonded to teeth to enhance and restore function and/or appearance. Veneers can be used to treat chipped, worn, crooked, and/or discolored teeth.
Walking bleach	A procedure to lighten a tooth that has darkened. The darkening can occur as a result of trauma and/or root canal treatment. A medicine is placed inside the tooth via the opening made for the root canal.
Wax pattern	A wax form that is made to resemble a tooth or a partial denture that is then cast in metal.
Whitening	The process of lightening discolored or stained teeth. Treatment can be in-office or at-home.
Wisdom tooth	These are the last teeth to erupt into the mouth and they usually appear around the age of 18, which is the reason for their name. Wisdom teeth are often impacted (obstructed from erupting), and are usually extracted.
Watt	Power measurement of energy produced over time.

Index

C

D

E

F

G

H

I

J

K

L

M

N

O

P

Q

R

S

T

U

V

W

X

Y

Made in the USA
Monee, IL
04 November 2026

67385371R00120